Praise for

Expecting Miracles

"Every physician and patient should read this book to learn the value of love, hope, faith, desire, intention; subjects which are not a normal component of medical education but which are important for healing and living a fertile life."

—Bernie Siegel, M.D.,

author of *Love, Medicine & Miracles*, and *Prescriptions for Living*

"Recognizing that undergoing fertility procedures can be an emotional roller-coaster ride for couples, Zouves carefully walks readers through the day-by-day, choice-by-choice process of battling infertility."

—*The Advocate*

"This testament to the pain of infertility and the promise of reproductive technology relentlessly accentuates the positive even as it describes the utter desperation of couples who are willing to do whatever it takes to have a child. . . . [Zouves] does an excellent job of recounting the physical, emotional, and financial toll that infertility treatment can take on his patients and their families. . . . For those grappling with infertility, Zouves' work, which makes the intricacies of biology understandable to the lay reader, offers a useful primer on cutting-edge science."

—*Kirkus Reviews*

"Upbeat, lively, and free of unnecessary technical terms."

—*Booklist*

Expecting Miracles

On the Path of Hope
from Infertility to Parenthood

Christo Zouves, M.D.
with Julie Sullivan

A Perigee Book

P

A Perigee Book
Published by The Berkley Publishing Group
A division of Penguin Group (USA) Inc.
375 Hudson Street
New York, New York 10014

Henry Holt and Company, LLC edition: 1999
Perigee edition: September 2003

Perigee ISBN: 0-399-52927-6

Visit our website at www.penguinputnam.com

Library of Congress Cataloging-in-Publication Data

Zouves, Christo.
Expecting miracles: on the path of hope from infertility to parenthood/
Christo Zouves with Julie Sullivan.—1st ed.
p.   cm.
ISBN 0-8050-6046-4 (hb: alk. paper)
1. Infertility—Treatment—Miscellanea.   2. Infertility, Female—
Treatment—Miscellanea.   3. Human reproductive technology—
Miscellanea.   4. Fertilization in vitro, Human—Miscellanea.
5. Artificial insemination, Human—Miscellanea.   I. Sullivan,
Julie, date.   II. Title.
RG201.Z68   1999   99-18781
616.6'9206—dc21   CIP

Printed in the United States of America
10   9   8   7   6   5   4   3   2   1

This book is dedicated to all the parents and teachers without whom I would not have had the privilege of sharing the infertility journey with so many special patients.

Contents

Acknowledgments

To the patients who shared their stories throughout these pages: You gave of yourselves in order to help others like you. We are all inspired by your tenacity, your strength, and your dreams. I thank you for making this book possible.

Thank you my family: my mother, father, and sister and my intelligent, dynamic, and beautiful partner, Miriam. I love you and our children, Natasha and Marky.

To Victor Gomel, my mentor, friend, and confidant, thank you for your vision, integrity, and pursuit of excellence.

Thanks to my wonderful staff, especially Linda Attell, Pamela Seifried, Suzanne Duffy, Shelley Tarnoff, Frank Barnes, and Anna Hosford for their work on this book.

Thank you to Amelia Sheldon, Wendy Sherman, Andrée Abacassis, literary agent, and Michelle Howry, editior, Perigee Books. I appreciate your faith in me.

None of this would have been possible without Mary Windishar Nickell, my publicist and friend, whose energy, editing, and experience as an infertility patient propelled this project forward.

And finally, a very special thank you to Julie Sullivan who saw the heroism and hope in every story and whose reporting and writing brought them to life. And to your family, Jim, Joe, and Rose Sullivan-Springhetti.

Foreword

It doesn't really matter whether the desire to have a child is socially conditioned or genetically hard-wired into us. The bottom line is that many people want to have children and many want genetically related children in particular. For those who experience difficulty in conceiving or in carrying a pregnancy to term, the desire for a child can be overwhelming and the pain of each failed attempt can be excruciating. Menstruation is monthly evidence of dashed hopes. Anything that reminds them of their childlessness can open the gaping wounds. Whether they show it or hide it, anguish and despair can fill their lives.

Dr. Christo Zouves, a physician who specializes in assisted reproduction and the treatment of male and female infertility, is all too familiar with the poignant stories of his patients' efforts to generate children. In *Expecting Miracles*, he shares many of their sagas with his readers. He tells us about their dreams, their sacrifices, their courage, their fortitude, their response to failures, and about the ultimate rewards that many are able to achieve with the help of reproductive medicine. Dr. Zouves also tells us a great deal more.

Until just a few decades ago, and for hundreds of years before that, assisted reproduction was a childless woman taking a lover with the intention of improving her chances of conception. That approach had its successes, but it also carried serious psychological, economic, and ethical risks. New technology improves the likelihood of reproductive success by identifying and addressing a far greater range of infertility problems. The new technology also raises a host of significant emotional, financial, and moral issues for those who consider its use. By mixing the narratives of real people with clear and thoughtful discussion of the problems they confront, *Expecting Miracles* introduces the reader to the full spectrum of issues that are raised by the new technology. While presenting his patients' stories, Dr. Zouves explains theoretical issues at points where such information is crucial for decision making. In this way, we are introduced to questions about embryo donation, post-menopausal reproduction, surrogacy, lesbian reproduction, cloning, pregnancy reduction, cancer, and social or familial reproductive relations. The natural motivation for these discussions makes the theorizing a compelling part of the narrative. Dr. Zouves's approach always communicates the sense that the issues his patients face are part of the fabric of human life rather than mere events in the realm of science fiction.

Dr. Zouves handles his presentation of complex information about reproductive biology and techniques for assisted reproduction in a similar way. The readers' need to understand guides the presentation of the biological and technical facts and makes them part of the story. So, as we read these very personal tales, we also learn a good deal about GIFT, ICSI, the relation of age to male and female infertility, hormones, antibodies, chromosomal abnormalities, activating sperm, and freezing and thawing embryos.

Dr. Zouves also weaves the history of advances in the understanding of reproductive biology and developments in reproductive technology into the personal accounts. In a way that adds richness and texture to the book, Dr. Zouves helps the reader appreciate the complex, cooperative process of scientific investigation and the rapid pace of recent technological developments. In many stories we are told about scientific advances that allow doctors to diagnose and treat problems such as the management of polycystic ovaries and ovarian hyperstimulation that would not have been understood just a few years ago. In other stories, we are told about technology that was not available when his patients needed it but can now help people with the same problem. We also learn about the contributions of leaders in the field such as Drs. Victor Gomel, Robert Edwards, Patrick Steptoe, Frank Barnes, Alan Trouson, Geoffrey Sher, and Victor Knutzen and about landmark events in the history of assisted-reproductive technology, such as the birth of Louise Brown in 1978, the first child engendered by in-vitro fertilization, and the birth of Elizabeth Carr shortly thereafter, the first IVF baby born in the United States.

And then there are the intimate details of personal experience. Dr. Zouves shares features of his own biography, specific aspects of some patients' experiences, and precise information about the experience of various treatments in the repertoire of reproductive medicine. He tells us about the cost of treatments, insurance realities, the frequency of injections, side effects of therapies, the position of the patient's body in various procedures, the telephone calls bringing good or bad news, some of the disabilities that can affect children, and the phenomenon of maternal love that sometimes comes at first sight and sometimes takes a few days longer. As in drama, these details enable those who have shared the experience to recall their own ordeals and they allow those who have no personal knowledge to empathize with the characters of Dr. Zouves's tales and to appreciate their suffering and their joy. And they enable those who are considering the use of reproductive technology to vividly imagine the experience and make more informed choices in that light.

By detailing his own responses to his patients' need for reproductive medicine, Dr. Zouves also shows that reproductive medicine is part of a medical tradition with implicit moral commitments. Through his own examples, he clearly conveys his view of a medical professional's responsibilities. We learn that physicians who practice reproductive medicine must be knowledgeable and skilled in their field; must provide all of the information that is relevant to their patients' choice so that those choices can reflect the patients' own values and priorities; must care a great deal about their patients' good and express that concern in their responsiveness and in compassionate, honest communication; and must be respectful of life choices and tolerant of patient values that may be different from their own. In sum, Dr. Zouves's attitudes offer a code of medical ethics, a standard that should constrain and guide every good physician's behavior.

Expecting Miracles informs us of important facts about reproduction and assisted-reproductive technology. It shows us how tremendously important having a child can be to some individuals. And it provides us with important lessons about the relationships that exist in families and between doctors and their patients. Christo Zouves is a compelling teacher and storyteller. I also believe that he must be a wonderful doctor.

Rosamond Rhodes, Ph.D.
Director of Bioethics Education
Mount Sinai School of Medicine

Introduction:
The Pressure of Life

*T*he yearning of human beings to have a family must be one of the most powerful forces in life.

The biological urge to perpetuate our genes, to see something of ourselves in our children, has propelled human evolution. To pass on characteristics through inheritance seems as much a Darwinian mandate as it is an emotional desire. It is the nature of living things to reproduce.

"If there are living beings on earth today it is because other beings have reproduced with desperate eagerness for two thousand million years," wrote the Nobel laureate Francois Jacob in *The Logic of Life*. "Let us imagine an uninhabited world."

Children are the projection of ourselves into the future. They are our bridge to adulthood. Parenthood is the ultimate rite of passage, an experience that, for many, completes the life experience. Having children is what we do when we grow up. We might have children for our parents' sake. They are our gift to our forebears. In a larger sense, it's our contribution to our society. Children are the building blocks of the nation. Children also can be a bridge to redemption. We might want children to re-create the family in which we grew up or, perhaps, to create the family we wished we had. They are our purest expression of love for another human being. The oldest form of valentine. The desire to have children is so elemental, so basic, and so natural that for most people the journey to parenthood begins with a single kiss.

The patients who walk through the doors of Zouves Fertility Center to meet me are successful people. They run companies, write laws, oversee real estate transactions, build businesses, orchestrate deals, and lead orchestras. They supervise classrooms, write press releases, produce television programs, and argue before judges. They counsel the mentally ill and treat the counselors. They operate on people. They believe that if you want something badly enough and work at it long enough and believe in yourself enough, you can get it. They are in control of their careers, their households, their time, and every aspect of their lives. Except their fertility.

By the time they reach me, they have stepped across a line as obvious as a border checkpoint. They are infertile and they have likely exhausted other surgical and pharmacological approaches and every popular suggestion. They've tried going on vacation and "just relaxing." They've drunk good wine.

It's a life crisis by the time we meet. These are healthy people seeking extensive medical intervention that cannot, in most cases, be considered a cure. In the prime of their lives, at the height of their personal, physical, intellectual, and earning powers, they need help. Their trust in their own bodies, their partner, and their belief in God or a higher power is often forever altered. Some blame themselves. They may have already lost a baby through miscarriage or stillbirth. What is wrong with me? they ask. Why me? Infertility is not a classic disease, but is affects people the same way disease does, emotionally and physically. It brings young, healthy people to the precipice of grief and loss.

The desire among physicians to help the infertile is as old as medicine itself. Hippocrates recognized infertility's singular anguish. *The Hippocratic Collection*, the writing of Hippocrates and Galen, which is the basis for all the medical studies of antiquity, devoted a whole book to sterile women. The chapters reveal the anxiety and concern of women unable to conceive or carry their pregnancies to term. Among the suggested treatments were vaginal suppositories and vaginal fumigation in the belief that fertility was based on good communication between the respiratory tract and the uterus.

More than twenty centuries later, in the last quarter of the twentieth century, medical science advanced enough to offer infertile couples real help. In vitro fertilization allows physicians to retrieve a woman's eggs, fertilize them outside the body, and successfully transfer a growing embryo back into the womb. Donated eggs, surrogacy, and the injection of a single sperm into an egg now overcome physical obstacles that prevented parenthood for thousands of years. Women who have gone through menopause can now mother; men with vasectomies can father; a woman without a uterus can have her own genetic child.

The dawn of the new millennium offers even greater hope with the introduction of Preimplantation Genetic Diagnosis. This intricate procedure which involves removing a single cell from a day three embryo and testing it for abnormalities, permits the selection of embryos, which are less likely to have chromosomal abnormalities and also embryos that may be free of a known single gene disorder, thereby increasing the likelihood of a healthy baby. This procedure is just the beginning of what's to come. The dominant driver and the new language of this century will be genetics. We will experience the genetics revolution as we experienced the digital revolution just a short time ago. The mapping of the human genome and applying this knowledge to the embryo will alter the way we practice IVF and the way humans reproduce. Soon IVF will be the means of having children for both the infertile and the fertile, and sex will just be for fun.

We must always remember that there is so much we do not know. We must recognize the limits of our view today and know that the techniques we rely on may appear tomorrow as primitive as the solutions the Greeks used thousands of years ago. The journey through in vitro fertilization is also one of scientific discovery. A journey that involves one single family at a time.

My life connects with those searching to create lives. It is no accident. On March 4, 1967, in my hometown of Kimberly, South Africa, my only brother, Spiro, cut a live electrical wire while playing on a walkie-talkie with a friend in an afternoon rain. He died instantly. He was twelve. I was fifteen. The grief in my parents' house was so raw and so deep that my mother believes it worked its way into my father's blood so that he died of leukemia within three years. Losing the two most important males in my life before I was eighteen set me on the journey that would eventually take me to San Francisco and my chosen profession, that of a physician and one specifically focused on helping infertile couples conceive children. I have felt every day since those losses the enormous pressure of life. Not to waste a single minute of it or to take it for granted. Life can, will, and every day does, end. Nothing is more precious, more central than to experience the present day and share it with those we love. Life itself is the miracle.

But many can't create life with those they love—millions of adults cannot have children. Together, they have created a number of international education and support groups that focus on specific aspects and treatment of infertility. These associations, and the emergence of the Internet, have empowered infertile women and men as never before, providing information and a sense of community. Through these channels many people find physicians as well. Like others in my field, I have my own Web address, www.GoIVF.com, which is how many patients are first introduced to me and my practice. Informal associations help as well, such as playgroups in California neighborhoods in which all the children were conceived in vitro. These connections help people take control of their problems and their choices. They help people feel less alone. Nevertheless, infertility is inevitably isolating. It singles people out. Each couple has a unique experience; it fills up their screen. What can comfort us, and caution us, is knowing what other people have experienced.

The following are the true stores of couples who've made the journey through in vitro fertilization in an attempt to have families. They begin the journey with no clear direction, no road map, and ultimately, no guarantee. The fear they face, the faith that sustains them, and the courage with which they proceed are testimony to the power of love and to the power of life, to the enormous pressure that we all feel, which has propelled the species through the eons.

It is my great, good fortune to have accompanied them along the way.

—Christo Zouves

Expecting Miracles

1 Dream Babies

Dream babies come when you call them. They've been waiting. Waiting all your life, in the movie picture that's been running in your head since childhood. Waiting for the right time, for the cue, for you to say, "It's time, Baby. We're ready. It's time." And they slide into the frame, into the present, in baby blankets and pink lotion, small and whole; and you hold them until your empty arms no longer ache.

Then, in the silence of an empty house, you wake up.

Kate* would wake up freezing, knees to chest, shivering in the heat and humidity of Florida. The fertility drugs she had swallowed five days in a row had turned on an internal faucet, drenching her with night sweats, making her head pound and her breasts sore. When she closed her eyes, she saw flashing lights and she felt so depressed, so contracted, that she could not unfold, get out of bed, and go into the warmth.

---

*The people whose stories are told in this book are real. But because of the sensitive nature of fertility issues and patient-doctor confidentiality, all names have been changed to protect patients and their families.

Other mornings she'd wake up praying, "Please God, let them find something wrong." Something identifiable—treatable—beyond what the doctor said was the reason she could not become pregnant.

The doctor said that she was tense. Tense.

Kate didn't know a single other person who couldn't have a baby. She grew up on the East Coast, a student of history and Spanish who took a right turn into nursing where the jobs were more secure. She met a tall New England doctor named Andy at a Christmas party when she was working at Massachusetts General as a cardiac intensive care nurse. Within a year, they were married and living in Florida. Their marriage was a twenty-four-hour-a-day honeymoon when, after eighteen months, they started trying to have children. Years passed. Kate didn't conceive. That's when she woke up.

She and Andy took every line of attack, from the first—clomiphene— to the last—in vitro fertilization. Day after day, Kate would crack open the ampules of fertility drugs for injections. They'd take the long flights to the best in vitro fertilization clinics she could find in the Northeast. Eighteen eggs were retrieved the first time and as many the second time; eggs round with hope. They were fertilized and the best transferred. She lost every one.

One doctor said Kate was preventing herself from getting pregnant. Another said she and Andy were overachievers who, for the first time in their lives, couldn't get what they wanted. Kate's family, which included several doctors, was silent. The relatives who could advise her on every other medical problem could not help in this arena. It was difficult for Kate not to feel like Don Quixote. It was difficult not to feel like a fraud as a woman.

Kate developed a radar for pregnant women. They were everywhere, setting off her private alarm. When Andy said he'd met a couple he'd like to see socially, she asked first, "Do they have kids?" If they did, the date was off. She walked away. She could not face that they had what she might never have: children.

She tried to swim away, too. Every day Kate would swim one full hour as fast and hard as she could, then move onto the stair-stepping machine, pushing her body while her mind raced to the next plan of attack. She and Andy did four in vitro cycles in one year. All the pregnancy results: negative. In the grief that followed, Andy would hold her, begging Kate to stop. "This is ruining our lives," he said. "It's tearing us apart."

Kate would plead to try one more time. She told Andy she had heard of a fertility clinic in San Francisco whose patients included women with numerous failed in vitro fertilization attempts. The doctors there had found that some of these women had antibodies that the doctors thought may be contributing to their infertility. Kate had her blood drawn, then sent to a Chicago laboratory that specialized in antibodies. The laboratory telephoned with the results: negative on the antibodies.

And then, a breakthrough. An adoption attorney Kate and Andy had contacted months before called with the best news the couple had heard in four years. A soon-to-be born baby girl was available for them to adopt. Baby Mary came to them the day she was born. It was the summer of 1993. Andy and Kate adored their adopted daughter and envisioned a whole family of Marys. The attorney indicated they were lucky to get Mary and not to count on adopting again any time soon. But they wanted more children, they wanted a houseful.

Then one morning, Kate was looking through a cluttered desk when she came across a copy of the antibody test results from the Chicago laboratory and examined it closely. She practically screamed. The lab had made a mistake in the telephone notification. She had tested positive for antiphospholipid antibodies. Kate picked up the telephone and called my office in San Francisco.

In vitro fertilization is the final common pathway when less aggressive approaches to infertility fail. On the western edge of that pathway is Zouves Fertility Center, which sits two stories up overlooking South San Francisco. The San Francisco Airport is five minutes away. In that clinic, my office is the last door on the left. This is where I meet the couples who have been trying so hard to conceive.

In the waiting room, Kate and Andy suddenly feel conspicuous sitting in a fertility center's lobby with baby Mary sucking her fingers on their laps. People are staring at them, and Kate recognizes the look instantly: part envy, part resentment.

"We adopted her," Kate explains to the other patients. "Ohhhh," the other couples say, starting to smile and relax. "Congratulations."

When Kate and Andy come into my office, they're veterans on the fertility front lines. They've had eight failed artificial inseminations, six failed in vitro fertilization cycles, two failed gamete intrafallopian transfers, and one cycle with a surrogate that failed the previous fall. Their diagnosis so far: "unexplained infertility."

When there is a clear reason why a couple cannot have a baby, because of a damaged tube or a low sperm count, we can tackle the problem and go on. But that isn't the case for the 5 percent of patients whose infertility is unexplained. There is a reason why they cannot conceive, of course; it's just beyond our understanding at this time. But the label "unexplained infertility" is like the sword of Damocles hanging over a patient's head, creating a suspended state of pain and anticipation. Many patients, if they just had an explanation for their infertility, could move on. Without one, their lives are spent searching. Why can't they have a baby? This is what they want to know.

Kate is young, just thirty-five, and when she takes fertility drugs, her ovaries make lots of eggs. More eggs mean more embryos, and more embryos give us the best chance of picking the best ones, including the one that will survive a transfer, implant, and grow into a healthy baby. Andy's sperm is normal. In other words, this couple has the basic ingredients for conception, but something is interfering with implantation.

Kate's blood tests revealed that she has antibodies that may either prevent the embryo from developing or cause clotting in the blood vessels that supply the early placenta, thus causing a miscarriage. This is the one clue we have. We have known since the late 1980s that women with high levels of antiphospholipid antibodies are more likely to have recurrent miscarriages. The risk of miscarriage dropped dramatically when doctors began using two common blood thinners, heparin and aspirin, for these patients. These prescriptions have been shown to prevent blood clots from forming in the blood vessels of the developing placenta. In the early 1990s, we began to extrapolate and use this treatment for women with repeated failed in vitro fertilization.

But this is not the only path Kate and Andy can take to pursue a pregnancy. We have three options. We can have them try for a spontaneous pregnancy while giving Kate heparin and aspirin. We can try using heparin and aspirin during an in vitro fertilization cycle. Or we can be really aggressive, and use a surrogate.

Andy and Kate have borrowed nearly $200,000 and spent five years attempting to have a baby. Financially, emotionally, and spiritually, they are almost wiped out. This ninth attempt cannot be a trial run. Until now, the couple's embryos have failed to implant. We can try improving the odds in Kate's favor, but we can also provide an alternative, a gestational surrogate. If we were to act most aggressively, we would transfer the couple's embryos into another woman whose uterus and immune system may be better able to support the embryos. Both women would receive embryos in the hopes of getting one or, at most, two babies. The risk, of course, is that both women could wind up pregnant.

By the time I raise the options open to them, Kate and Andy have already made the decision to try using both Kate and a surrogate. Kate is willing to undergo another attempt, but is skeptical of her chances. As much as she would like to believe what I tell her about immunology, she has used the blood thinner heparin on patients throughout her nursing career. She knows it is not a magic potion. On the basis of their history, both she and Andy hope that the surrogate will become pregnant. Now they just have to find one.

After Kate and Andy leave my office, they contact a California agency that helps locate surrogates. The agency finds Jan, a thirty-year-old woman who lives one town away from Kate and Andy in Florida. Jan flies to San Francisco to complete the physical and psychological testing required by our center before she will ever meet the couple with whom she may be working very closely. Her husband also consults with our staff psychologist over the telephone.

Several weeks later, the doorbell rings at Kate and Andy's home in Florida. Kate peeks out the window, and there standing on the porch is a woman wearing a long, flowing, flowered dress that reaches almost to her ankles. She is very pretty and very feminine. The goddess of fertility, Kate thinks. It's Jan.

Jan is married with one daughter. She was adopted as an infant herself and had grown up with a powerful insight into infertility from hearing her mother talk about her struggle before adopting Jan. For reasons she almost can't explain, Jan wants to help a couple by being a surrogate. It's the ultimate gift and, in some ways, is giving back to the world some of the generosity that people showed her.

As motivated as Jan is, walking up to the door of complete strangers to discuss having their baby is no easy thing. For Kate, neither is opening that door. But the two women instantly connect. They start talking and four weeks later, in late January 1994, when they fly to San Francisco with Andy and baby Mary, they are still talking.

My challenge is to synchronize both women's cycles so that each woman's uterus is prepared for the embryos that result from Kate's eggs and Andy's sperm. At home in the weeks before they come to San Francisco, both women take birth control pills, bringing their cycles into perfect synch. Then, Kate takes fertility drugs and hormones to prepare her uterus, while Jan, the surrogate, receives the hormones natural estrogen and progesterone.

Earlier, after seeing the results of some tests, I had worried that Kate's ovaries are becoming resistant to the fertility drugs. But her ovaries respond beautifully. I am able to retrieve eighteen eggs, which are mixed with Andy's sperm in the laboratory. Fifteen embryos result. Three days later, Andy and the two women come in for the embryo transfers. Baby Mary is with them. She sits, wearing a pink romper, in a stroller between the two women. Kate reaches out frequently to touch the baby, and it feels strange to her to be doing all this "fertility stuff" when she already has a child. But she believes that Mary and Andy, the people she loves the most, will benefit for the rest of their lives from another child. In addition, she is still the woman she has been the last five years. She is a woman on a quest.

After a discussion, I transfer six of the healthiest-looking embryos into Jan and nine poorer embryos into Kate. As I discuss in chapter 13, embryos are graded prior to transfer. Poorer-quality embryos do not make poor-quality babies, of course; they just aren't as likely to survive and implant. The transfers go well.

Throughout their many treatments, Andy would draw Kate's blood for the pregnancy tests and deliver it to the local hospital laboratory personally. Both he and his wife got very used to bad news from the hospital staff. When a staff member calls them this time to report that Kate is pregnant, Kate makes Andy call the hospital lab back—twice. Then they call me in San Francisco. Kate and Jan are both pregnant.

Jan is thrilled, and Kate is ecstatic. The women begin meeting in a home improvement store parking lot halfway between their homes so that Kate can give Jan a shot or draw blood or just so that they can get together to talk and have lunch nearby.

Kate tells Jan the most unpleasant aspect of the medications are the golf-ball-sized bruises on her tummy and hips from the injections.

Heparin must be injected every twelve hours into the fatty tissue of the tummy or hips with a short, thin needle. Getting the injection doesn't hurt as much as it hurts to look at the bruises that result. Kate, like most women in her situation, begins taking the medication in the week before the embryo transfer and expects to continue the injections for twelve weeks. Because the blood thinner is most concentrated at the injection site, the bruises around the navel area are substantial. But, Kate says, she would gladly do this and more if it means she might have a baby after all.

Then, on February 7, the level of pregnancy hormones in Kate's blood abruptly drops, then disappears. There is no apparent cause. She and Andy have that old visit with grief once again. The blood, and then the tears. Their consolation is that Jan is pregnant and carrying their baby.

However, the image on the monitor at Jan's ultrasound at six weeks quiets that joy, as well. There is no heartbeat. The second week of March Jan begins bleeding; she has cramps and passes tissue. Both pregnancies are lost. I'm stunned. Kate, Andy, and Jan are devastated.

Amid the grief, there is guilt. Kate has created more than sixty-five embryos and a potential baby in the course of her fertility treatment. In her eyes, her body has killed every one of them. She tells me she feels like her face should be on the post office wall with other criminals. She's the embryo killer, the woman who destroys life. Jan feels her own grief and guilt that she has let this couple down. She's come to love Kate and Andy, and she reaches a decision. She says that if Kate needs her eggs—the genetic material she said she'd never part with—she would gladly donate them to her, with blessings.

Kate and Andy's friends and colleagues, meanwhile, are openly skeptical about the treatment the couple is pursuing. In 1994, few clinics nationally were taking immunology into account when it came to infertility, and more than one professional called the treatment I had prescribed for them "voodoo medicine."

Kate calls me, emotionally exhausted, and tells me she would like to end her treatment, stop the torture.

I told her that she has had the worst luck of anyone I've ever treated, but that I truly believed there was hope. I encouraged her to consider one last attempt.

People come here to have a baby. My job is to explain the means available to them and to try to give them my best medical estimation of what their chances of having a baby would be with a particular treatment. I constantly reinforce that they have a spectrum of choices. I urge them to take control and make decisions. I try to restore some of the power that so many feel they have lost in pursuit of fertility.

Kate and Jan have become pregnant, however briefly. What was the last of many devastating blows to Kate and Andy was, to me, a glimpse of light. This is why I suggested a tenth cycle.

When I was an intern in Capetown, South Africa, there was an old doctor I watched closely. If a patient had a heart attack, the doctor would go to the family and say, "You know, this is the worst heart attack I've ever seen in my life." If the patient died, well, the family accepted it. It was, after all, the worst heart attack the doctor had ever seen. If the patient lived, the doctor was like God, because he had saved this man from the worst heart attack.

In this way the old doctor built the biggest practice in town. I believe his success was intellectually and ethically a scam. Any doctor, like the one I've mentioned, can protect himself by painting the bleakest picture and then emerge the hero if the outcome is favorable. But doing so robs patients of the accurate picture they should have of their chances with a particular treatment. I am a realist, and I want my patients to know the truth of their situation. But I am also an optimist, and if there is hope, I want the couple to know. While there is no way to measure the power of such intangibles, my opinion is that they can affect the outcome of many medical procedures. I always want my patients to have hope on their side.

If a couple knows and understands that they are pursuing treatment with a 10 percent chance of success, it's my mandate to give 100 percent of my support to that fraction of hope and not remind them of the 90 percent chance of failure.

Kate and Andy have a real chance. They don't need Jan's eggs. Kate continues to make beautiful follicles and eggs. But we need to address the implantation problem. I'm going to keep Kate on heparin and aspirin, and I think with another attempt, we can make this happen. They decide to try one more time.

On their first trip to my office, Kate, Andy, and Jan spent a leisurely ten days in San Francisco. This cycle, on the other hand, is the equivalent of a drive-by. Andy flies into San Francisco to produce a sperm sample and leaves just as Jan is arriving. On June 12, they have twelve embryos from Kate. After careful discussion with Kate and Andy, I direct the laboratory staff to divide the embryos. Kate and Andy decide that the best and healthiest-appearing ones should be transferred to Jan. They believe she will have the best chance for becoming pregnant.

As soon as their required hour of rest following the transfers is over, the two women take none of the careful and restful steps they did previously. They jump up, dress as quickly as possible, and rush downstairs to catch a cab. They zoom to the airport and run twenty gates to catch their plane back to Florida. They don't stop hurrying until after takeoff.

Both Kate and Jan agreed that if anything took after all that, it would be a miracle.

It is a miracle. It is multiple miracles.

In their first blood tests upon returning home, the level of pregnancy hormones in both women is rising steeply, with Kate's rising faster. Kate puts down the phone after receiving the news and thinks that, after six years of bloody all-out war, she's won.

At six weeks an ultrasound confirms Kate is carrying twins. So is Jan. In fact, there are three gestational sacs with two heartbeats visible on her sonogram. After the sonogram, Jan is ravenous, and the two women drive to McDonald's for lunch. But the smell of frying food suddenly makes them both a little nauseated. Kate is in shock. She can't speak. All of a sudden it hits her: five babies. All she can think of is five babies.

But nature steps in and reabsorbs two of the three gestational sacs Jan is carrying. By the time they leave my care at twelve weeks, Jan is pregnant with one baby. And, Kate, who had nine failed cycles and received the embryos least likely to implant and grow, is pregnant with two. It's a small distinction, but the woman who believed for so long that she wasn't a real woman just lapped the goddess of fertility.

Postscript

After two and a half months on bedrest, Kate delivered twins at thirty-five weeks, a five pound, five ounce boy and a four pound, eleven ounce girl. Three weeks to the day later, she stood at Jan's side as Jan delivered the third triplet, another girl, at seven pounds, eleven ounces. Seeing the looks on Kate's and Andy's faces was one of the high points of Jan's life. She only wished it wasn't over so soon.

Having four small children turned Andy and Kate's world upside down. Some days Kate wishes she could clone herself, a wish shared by parents everywhere. She has permanent nerve damage in her hips from the fertility drug shots; if she bumps a countertop wrong, she feels a sharp jolt. The stress of the last ten years has taken its toll. Andy spends a lot of time making sure Mary gets plenty of attention. And Kate delights that out of all her children her adopted daughter looks the most like her. The triplets hardly slow down to enable one to compare them to Mary or one another.

Jan stays in touch and occasionally comes to visit. Her own daughter has stayed with Kate for the night. It takes a while to get everyone settled at bedtime, in sleepers and with blankies and four old teddy bears. Bedtime may be Kate's favorite time of all. When the dream babies are home, safe and asleep.

2 *Life Lessons*

Graham had had enough. Two months waiting for the doctor's appointment, two hours sitting in a hardback chair, the minute hand flicking forward like a mosquito . . . enough. Enough of the probing and the plastic cups and the scheduled sex and the dye injected into his wife's fallopian tubes until she'd almost fainted and more than enough waiting. For blood test results to come back from the laboratory. For doctors to report them. For the paid professionals to tell them what was obvious: They couldn't get pregnant.

"Have you got a watch?" he says. "Because if you don't have a watch, I can buy you a watch. If you need a watch, I'll get you a watch. But I can't be sitting here all day waiting for you."

I extend my hand. "Doctor Zouves."

"Businessman Jones," he retorts in the flat, clipped speech of a Newcastle man. He and his wife, Linda, had been waiting a long time. Years, really. When they arrive at the University of British Columbia in Vancouver in 1985, the waiting list for fertility treatment is three years long. The office visit they had waited months for is being squeezed into my schedule between high-risk pregnancies and faculty duties at the medical school, between surgeries, tutorials, research, rounds, late nights, and long weekends all subject to the unplannable, unknowable schedule of arriving babies. It's Monday. I'd been working since Friday and had been up all night with a birth. But this schedule isn't fair to them. They need my full attention.

Linda and Graham have been together since he spotted her at a dance in Newcastle Upon Tyne, a girl taller and more willowy than the others. She had gray-green eyes. He asked her for a dance and then for a kiss because, he said, it was his twentieth birthday. He was lying. She kissed him anyway, forgave him, and married him shortly after in a northeast English city a dozen miles from the North Sea. When he was hired by a petroleum company in Toronto, Canada, they packed everything they owned into a few bags and immigrated. By the time they relocated a decade later to Vancouver, on the west coast of Canada, it took a moving van to transport the household.

They'd wanted a child, and they had one, a fair-haired boy. They wanted another, for themselves, to re-create what they'd experienced as parents, and for their son. For him to have a sibling, a lasting connection in a transient world.

None came. They tried for months and then years. They tried predicting ovulation, timing sex, using ovulation drugs and artificial insemination. They assumed they were the same people they had been five years earlier but came to understand they were not. They've come here to the university's Division of Infertility and Reproductive Endocrinology for help. Canada's first in vitro baby had been born through the program two years earlier in 1983. I'm the doctor directing the program and, therefore, the object of Graham's disaffection.

Linda and Graham are experiencing secondary infertility, the inability to conceive after a couple has already had a biological child together. The cause is likely a condition that has developed since their son was born, or an underlying cause that has become worse since his birth.

Whatever it is, in order for the three of us to decide what to do about it, we'll need Graham's full support first. In fertility medicine, the doctor-patient relationship is the doctor-couple relationship. The decisions are too difficult and the consequences for the entire family too great for the discussion to be exclusively between the intended mother and me, the doctor. So although Graham would like to take my head off, at this moment, after all the waiting, we have to try to get along. The dearest thing in his life, his wife, is about to go through a major medical procedure, and he needs to be involved and know what to expect.

I don't know why they haven't been able to conceive. Linda is thirty-three. She appears to have healthy fallopian tubes, and Graham's sperm is normal. The inexplicable nature of their dilemma makes her a candidate for GIFT, gamete intrafallopian transfer. The procedure, developed at the University of Texas in San Antonio the year before, in 1984, is being offered for the second time in North America to patients in Vancouver. The process involves using fertility drugs to stimulate Linda's ovaries to produce eggs and then retrieving the eggs using a laparoscope, a telescope-like instrument that allows us to view the internal organs. The eggs would be placed in a petri dish with Graham's sperm for about ten minutes, then transferred into a catheter and immediately injected into Linda's fallopian tubes during the same laparoscopic procedure. The idea is that sheer numbers of sperm and eggs and the natural and nurturing environment of the woman's body will overcome subtle or unexplained obstacles preventing a pregnancy.

It's been seven years since the world's first "test tube" baby was born, but Linda and Graham feel no earthly connection to her or the technology her birth heralded. To them, assisted reproduction is common sense, a mechanical shortcut to solving a problem. It appeals to both of them.

"Physically, chemically, organically, statistically, it all makes sense," Graham says when the intervention is described. They join almost forty families who have signed up for the experimental GIFT treatment in the provincial medical system. The cost to them, not including medication, will be $750.

Introducing Graham and Linda to the concept of in vitro fertilization makes me remember the first time I was in an in vitro laboratory. At thirty-three, I'd already trained and worked as an obstetrician and gynecologist and surgeon in England and South Africa. When I immigrated to Canada, I worked as a family practitioner, then completed my specialist certification in obstetrics and gynecology. For years I'd met patients who'd been trying to have a baby. There wasn't a lot we could do for them. I had just finished additional training in infertility and reproductive endocrinology when I got a call from Reno, Nevada.

There was an opportunity to join two of my former medical school professors who had opened the fourth in vitro fertilization clinic in the United States in Reno. Drs. Geoffrey Sher and Victor Knutzen opened Northern Nevada Fertility, the first in vitro center to operate outside a university setting. The first IVF baby in United States had been born just three years earlier, Elizabeth Carr of Virginia. The techniques, information, and vision Sher and Knutzen shared with me on the in vitro process were invaluable.

I will never forget seeing assisted reproduction for the first time. It was amazing to see the union of sperm and egg outside the body. To look through a microscope eighteen hours later and see twin craters on the egg, the two pronuclei, that indicate fertilization has taken place. Seeing the two polar bodies, small bubbles on the egg that look like lights on a police cruiser. The polar bodies hold the twenty-three chromosomes discarded from each parent while inside the egg the twenty-three pairs of chromosomes from the mother have fused with the twenty-three from the father. All the potential for a unique individual is right there.

To watch as, within three days, the single fertilized cell becomes two and then four and then eight-celled embryos could be transferred into a woman. (Cells do not divide at the same minute, so it is possible to have six cells for a time until the other divides.) To know the woman could and did become pregnant. For me, seeing that was like standing at an Apollo launch. I was on the edge of exploration and space.

But I never moved to Reno. My green card application moved through U.S. immigration at such a glacial pace that I was offered a full-time faculty position at the University of British Columbia in the interim. I was offered an opportunity to direct the department's disorganized in vitro program, to work with patients and conduct research under the chairmanship of Professor Victor Gomel. It was a chance I could not pass up. Gomel is one of the key figures in the treatment and hope offered infertile couples.

In 1972, the young Canadian gynecologist Victor Gomel heard an English geneticist speak at the Athens Hilton. Professor Robert Edwards presented a paper on human eggs and his technique to fertilize them outside the body and allow them to divide and grow. Afterward, as Gomel would come to tell me, he and Edwards had a beer together, and Gomel learned more in that hour than he had during the entire conference. The potential for retrieving eggs, fertilizing them outside the body, and returning the embryo to the uterus set his mind racing. This new procedure meant that for the first time women with blocked and damaged fallopian tubes could become pregnant. Listening to Edwards, Gomel realized that the future he was discussing depended on a good laboratory, a place embryos could survive and grow. Gomel asked Edwards if he would consider training an individual for a lab at the University of British Columbia and Edwards said, "Of course." But the Canadians were not ready to embrace the concept.

Within six years, Edwards successfully teamed up with a gynecologist and skilled handler of the laparoscope, Dr. Patrick Steptoe of Oldham, England. The team retrieved, fertilized, and transferred a single embryo that became the world's first in vitro fertilization baby in 1978. Shortly afterward, Gomel became chairman of the Department of Obstetrics and Gynecology at the University of British Columbia.

Gomel never forgot Edwards's vision. "Nothing happens without vision. Nothing happens without courage; nothing happens without effort," he would say.

As chairman, Gomel began in 1981 to put the in vitro fertilization program he envisioned in place, and on Christmas Day, 1983, a woman gave birth to Canada's first IVF baby, a boy. In spite of this success, the program died shortly after for lack of a designated director. There were no patients being treated when I took on reviving it as a project during my final subspecialty training. My mandate was to resurrect the program and reintroduce in vitro fertilization as an option for the infertile population of western Canada.

I approached this challenge with Gomel's help; he had the vision and ability to build consensus and to create the environment that makes it possible. He developed a safe haven for innovation to flourish. It was as obvious in the operating theater as it was in our efforts at assisted reproduction. For example, the laparoscope was developed around the turn of the century in Germany, but it was not widely used until Gomel and a handful of other gynecologists brought back the techniques from Europe and England in the early 1970s and revolutionized reproductive surgery.

Before that happened, almost all tubal, reproductive, or gynecological surgeries were laparotomies, major surgeries performed by opening the abdomen with a bikini incision—a horizontal incision above the pubic area—or a vertical incision. Women undergoing the procedure were in the hospital up to a week and were out of their usual activities for a month or more.

But the laparoscope allows surgeons to perform many of the same operations without making such long incisions in the abdomen. A small incision is made in or just below the navel, and the laparoscope is inserted. The doctor, wearing an eyepiece, can look through the long, thin, lighted telescope of the laparoscope to see the internal organs. Then, two to three additional puncture sites are made in the lower abdomen in order to insert probes, grasping instruments, and suturing materials. With this new, less-invasive technique, the patient requires less anesthetic, can go home in a day or two, and is able to resume most activity within a week. It's a diagnostician's dream. To be able to see inside the body and visually detect fibroids, endometriosis, and ectopic pregnancies. To treat pelvic disorders—such as removing cysts, fibroids, or diseased ovaries—without opening the abdomen.

Initially, even the procedure for gamete intrafallopian transfer was done through a mini-laparotomy or abdominal surgery, when Gomel suggested it could be done through the laparoscope. That step helped lead us to offer gamete intrafallopian transfer, or GIFT, in Canada.

Gomel spent much of his long career looking for ways to help infertile patients. In the 1970s, techniques known as microsurgery were developed to repair blood vessels. He again was among the first to apply these techniques to fertility patients.

"A lot of people don't view infertility as a disease. The attitude is, 'So, okay, you're not having children.' I remember this remarkable man saying, 'They don't see the stress and the anguish and frustration of people who cannot achieve it.'"

Gomel's influence in my life and my career will last a lifetime. My office was next door to his office at The Grace Hospital in Vancouver and over sandwiches, coffees, long days, and late nights, we discussed everything: the ethics of in vitro fertilization, technology, history, philosophy, finances, faith, and whether I should buy a condominium. It was a once-in-a-lifetime relationship with a teacher who became a brother and a father to me.

I learned much from Gomel on every level. I watched him step back from the emotional side of a case, then clearly and analytically synthesize the essence of a problem, and ultimately move toward a solution. It's a clinical, rational approach, and yet he is the last man anyone would call cold. It is simple balance, and balance is essential in the emotionally charged fields of obstetrics and gynecology and fertility treatment, a trip that most patients liken to riding a roller coaster.

In 1985, success rates for IVF patients were about 10 percent. Ninety percent of the women completed a cycle without delivering a baby. Even when all the variables seemed right, more often than not the procedure failed. When it worked, we thanked God.

"One must recognize that, irrespective of what you do, you don't make the patient pregnant. She gets pregnant," Gomel says. "Even if you put an advanced embryo like a blastocyst in the uterus, a pregnancy may not result. A lot of people fail in spite of heroic efforts. We can't control everything—that is very important for you and the patient to know ahead of time."

In the years I spent working with Gomel, advances in laparoscopy propelled a worldwide trend toward minimally invasive surgery. Laparoscopy would become the most frequently performed abdominal procedure in the world, used in everything from gynecological to general surgery. Together, we extended the scope of the less-invasive approach to include removing fibroids and ovarian cysts and treating ectopic pregnancies. Gomel is a perfectionist who demands as much of himself as a surgeon as he does his staff. But it's the instruction outside the operating theater that left a mark.

"What good is it to be a technician if you don't have the philosophy and humanity behind it?" he says.

Those words of my mentor Gomel cross my mind often in the case of Linda and Graham. Now, late in the summer of 1985, I am helping the couple prepare for a GIFT cycle.

Linda's eggs have been stimulated with fertility drugs and we are readying for the retrieval and transfer, which will be conducted during laparoscopic surgery. In my conference with Linda and Graham, Linda is quiet during a discussion about how many eggs to transfer. I tell this couple that there is a substantial risk of multiple pregnancy and ectopic pregnancy. Most clinics are transferring at least three to five eggs during the procedure in the hope that one will fertilize in the fallopian tube and implant. I tell them this, but Graham doesn't like the odds. He's calculated his chances of success based on the reported success rates, and he wants to inject six eggs or more. Linda is finding it difficult to see how any of this talk applies to her. She hasn't been able to conceive one child in six years and can't imagine getting pregnant with two. She ultimately agrees with her husband, opting for more than the customary number of eggs transferred.

I refuse to transfer more than six. We compromise on six, hoping that one will successfully implant and grow.

I begin the procedure with Linda under general anesthetic. Her tummy is inflated with carbon dioxide, and I insert the laparoscope into her abdomen and use the aspiration needle to get through to the ovary. I remove the eggs from the follicles and give them to an assistant to carry to the laboratory. The staff there identifies and grades them for maturity. The eggs are then mixed with Graham's sperm, put into a thin catheter, and I immediately reinject them into the fallopian tube through another incision. The whole procedure takes less than an hour.

"If this works, I owe you a case of champagne," Graham says afterward. "If it doesn't, you owe *me*." He voices the hope and applies the pressure that most of my patients feel at this point.

Linda telephones me a few days later. She's noticed some faint pink spotting and is worried. This may be good news—implantation bleeding—I tell her. A small percentage of pregnant women will bleed in the first trimester of pregnancy for this reason, as the early placenta begins to take hold in the uterine wall and hits a little blood vessel. It often seems to happen around the time of a positive pregnancy test. A blood test subsequently confirms that Linda is indeed pregnant and, based on the level of hormone in her blood, I'd guess that she's probably pregnant with more than one. In her first ultrasound we see that that is the case. Three embryo sacs are obvious in the uterus.

A delivery comes to the office one day, a case of Moët. I know immediately who it's from. I'm surprised to get such an extravagant gift but not surprised by the man who sent it. Graham is as good as his word.

Two weeks later Linda wakes with a shudder from a sound sleep. Pain presses through her abdomen like a giant auger grinding front to back.

She can't breathe, can't keep anything down. She calls to Graham; when he sees her gray with pain, he calls me.

I tell Graham to bring her into the hospital straightaway, and an ultrasound confirms my suspicions. Two embryo sacs are clearly visible in the uterus. Two others are growing in her right fallopian tube. Ectopic pregnancies similar to this one occur once in every one hundred spontaneous pregnancies, usually because of some abnormality in the fallopian tube. Some remain undetected, the embryo dies, and the tissue is reabsorbed before causing any symptoms. Others develop a placenta that continues to grow inside the tube as though the tube were the uterus. As it grows, the placenta invades the blood vessels in the tube, causing pain, swelling, tenderness, and ultimately, rupture and hemorrhage. The further along the rupture, the more catastrophic the result. Young healthy women still die from ectopic pregnancies.

Linda needs surgery immediately. She has been stoic in the face of extreme pain until she's asked to sign a consent to abdominal surgery. Then she starts to cry. "I'm going to lose my baby," she says. I tell her we're going to take her into surgery and do everything we can to prevent that.

Unfortunately, the hospital is being renovated, and the operating rooms are closed for a brief time while a new air-conditioning system is installed. I make arrangements to send Linda a few blocks by ambulance to a nearby Catholic hospital, and then I gather up my instruments including forceps, graspers, and scissors. I will sterilize them as soon as I arrive at the alternate site.

My first priority is immediately to get Linda out of pain and out of danger. To do that I'm going to attempt to treat the ectopic pregnancy using the laparoscope. By doing so I hope to cause the least amount of trauma to Linda's abdomen and therefore to maintain the pregnancy. This means going in through three or four small incisions instead of opening her abdomen with a major surgery.

To Graham the procedure seems about as easy as wallpapering the front hallway through the letter slot. I have operated on other women who have had both a uterine and tubal pregnancy. Although I'm concerned about saving the uterine pregnancy, my main priority is to complete this operation quickly before a fatal hemorrhage in Linda's fallopian tube begins.

Linda is prepped at the nearby hospital, and I soon join her in the operating room. I make the small incisions necessary and begin my exploration. Through the laparoscope I see the fallopian tube. One sac has implanted right toward the end, and I'm able to squeeze it out. The other is painfully obvious in the middle, and we have to remove it surgically and tie off the tube.

When Linda regains consciousness, she's distraught. A nurse, unaware of her uterine pregnancies, keeps trying to comfort her over her loss. The subsequent ultrasound, though, shows that she's still pregnant. The third and smallest sac we saw in the uterus weeks earlier has disappeared. Two other sacs appear large and obvious in the uterus, each with a heartbeat.

As soon as she can sit up, Linda calls England. Linda wants to share the good news with her mother, who needs it. "Mum," she says, "it's twins." Linda will forever remember the call and the joy in her mother's voice. Earlier that spring, her mother was diagnosed with lung cancer. Shortly after this phone conversation, Linda's mother enters a hospital on a public ward with no phone service. She dies before they ever speak again.

The ensuing months are bleak and depressing. Vancouver weather in winter is wet upon wet. Linda is home taking care of their son when she begins spotting again, heavily. I hospitalize her with placenta previa, a condition marked by the placenta being located low in the uterus, near or over the cervix. I explain that this condition is dangerous during the last trimester of pregnancy when there is a lot of stretching in preparation for the baby's head to come down. This stretching can pull or shear the placenta from the uterine wall. We must put Linda on bedrest to reduce the stress on the placenta. The sadness Linda feels over her mother and the guilt she feels over leaving her eldest child, Jonathan, to pursue another pregnancy are extreme. Feeling torn between a child already here in this world and the rigors of the treatment to have a second child is a division women with secondary infertility often face.

Over the weeks of bedrest, Linda and Graham's son, Jonathan, bounces from friend to friend, eating out with his father after work each night; they must have tried every restaurant in the city. Some weeks, if Graham is traveling and the boy is with friends, Linda goes days without seeing anyone but hospital staff. So after five weeks of bedrest, Linda is looking forward to going home, where she will continue to take it easy. She takes great care, drinking her milk, avoiding stairs and housework. Each night she smoothes oil onto the stretched skin of her tummy.

At twenty-nine weeks, settling down into bed with her husband one night at about 11:30 P.M., Linda feels a gush of warm fluid between her legs. Pulling back the bedcovers she almost chokes. All she sees is blood, dark red and clotted. This, she knows, is the end.

Graham grabs a bathrobe and brings towels to staunch the flow. He calls two friends to stay with their sleeping son. The boy is curled up in his bed, oblivious. By the time the couple leaves for the hospital, the mattress is so sodden it will have to be thrown away.

Calling from their car, they reach me at home to say they are headed to the local emergency room of a nearby suburban hospital.

I am thinking about what Graham is saying and considering the options. Linda is twenty-nine weeks into the pregnancy, a good seven weeks early. If Graham and Linda go into a small hospital, it's likely those babies will be delivered tonight and they'll have very fragile two-pound twins on their hands. I can almost hear my mentor Gomel say, "Step back."

"Do you think you can make it to The Grace Hospital in the city?" I ask. The hospital has one of the best high-risk obstetric wards in North America. If she delivers, the babies will be in the best possible hands. If she stabilizes, we may be able to buy the twins a few more days.

It is a tough call, because when somebody is bleeding, the safest thing is to get him or her to the nearest hospital. I am trying to gauge how much Linda has actually bled as well as the source of the blood, and Graham is driving like a madman, talking to me on the car phone, trying to convey the details that will help me determine the best plan. I tell them to try for Grace. I jump into my car and drive there to meet them.

I am outside the emergency room doors waiting with a gurney when Linda and Graham pull into the parking lot. Inside are a team of doctors and nurses and two acrylic incubators. Linda remembers hands reaching for her, pulling off her ruined dressing gown, starting intravenous lines. She is naked, her skin translucent, legs bloody, and she closes her eyes under the lights and motion around her. She lies there, so helpless, so utterly exposed that, for once, Graham has nothing to say. He goes outside, badly shaken.

The dilemma of obstetrics is timing: knowing when a baby will be better outside its mother's body than within. The placenta is starting to separate from the wall of Linda's uterus, as we had feared earlier. She has lost so much blood we'll have to give her two units intravenously. But the babies appear fine. They will still clearly benefit from remaining inside the uterus, as long as the bleeding stops. If we can get Linda's uterus to relax and stabilize, we may make it through the night. I find Graham outside, pacing, hunched against the cold.

"You should have seen the blood," he says. "It was just pouring out of her. It scared the hell out of me."

"I've seen it a lot, and it scares the hell out of me, too," I say. I am worried. Linda's placenta is beginning to pull away from the uterine wall, putting both the babies and her at risk. The placenta is their lifeline, and if the sac detaches, she can bleed to death and the babies would be lost. He asks me for the odds. There is probably only a 30 to 40 percent chance things will settle down and go the way we both pray they will. We agree that the next step is just to wait.

Linda makes it to the next morning. And the next. After a week of complete bedrest, she insists on getting up to go to the bathroom and eventually to a daily shower. She settles into the life of a sanatorium patient, like someone from the last century, spending her days reading in bed or being wheeled into the sunshine on the patio. Graham and Jonathan come at night to visit, and I find myself staying longer and longer on my nightly rounds, sitting and talking. This couple is full of wry humor and passion for the lives they've created on this side of the Atlantic. We enjoy our visits and are becoming good friends.

At thirty-six weeks, the condition of the babies begins to change. One baby seems to have stopped growing, and the other's growth is accelerated. The ultrasound shows low levels of amniotic fluid surrounding the smaller twin. It is time to welcome these babies into the world. We schedule a C-section under epidural on April 30, 1986. That day, Linda is quite afraid of the scalpel; she is lying there bracing for the slice in her abdomen when I say, "I'm lifting the first baby out. It's a girl."

Linda starts to cry. By the time baby number two is pulled out a minute later and I say, "It's a boy," she is sobbing, a tidal wave of hormones and raw relief so powerful that it awes the team of sixteen gathered in the room.

A doctor feels a rare completeness having been present at both the conception and the birth. I now see two heads, covered with jet-black hair, perfectly formed, two screaming mouths. I throw my arms around Graham, who's been sitting at Linda's head, holding her hand.

"You have two beautiful babies." A six pound, ten ounce boy and a five pound, fifteen ounce girl.

"Christ, they look like skinny little rabbits," says the Newcastle man. He is laughing, of course, and crying, and the photographs of those moments show perfect joy.

Postscript

When the sixth graders in a Pacific Northwest classroom began studying how babies are conceived and born, one twelve-year-old boy politely interrupted the teacher and said it hadn't worked that way at his house.

"A doctor took my mom's eggs and my dad's sperm and mixed them in a bowl and put them back, and then he cut her stomach open, a cesa . . . section . . . a cesarean section. Well, she had us."

"Cool," said one classmate.

"Gross," said another.

The boy recounted this story while sitting in a large and airy kitchen with his twin sister, eating turkey sandwiches, and looking out at the world with eyes the same color as the sea on a stormy day: gray-green.

"GIFT, I don't even know what that means," said Jonathan, the twins' twenty-year-old brother, as he walked into the kitchen.

"Basically, it means we're fake," said the twelve-year-old's twin sister.

"It means it was a team effort," said their mother, Linda.

The team effort made national news in Canada the year it took place.

Ironically, Gomel and I later published papers showing no advantage of GIFT over in vitro fertilization. For years the procedure was perceived to be more successful than in vitro fertilization, but two randomized studies, including ours and one in Norway, showed no statistical difference. GIFT requires general anesthetic and laparoscopy, and is more invasive than conventional IVF. I have not offered the procedure to my patients since 1990.

Gomel is still in Vancouver, a practicing surgeon and mentor whose former students now lead hospital programs and clinics around the world. He and his friend Robert Edwards, the father of in vitro fertilization, met again at a recent World Congress on assisted reproduction, where they were president and honorary president respectively.

I left Vancouver in 1992 to join Geoffrey Sher, who had moved to California from Reno and founded Pacific Fertility Center, San Francisco. The years in British Columbia gave me many practical skills in laparoscopic surgery, research, and the running of an in vitro program. I also stopped delivering babies in order to concentrate full-time on my fertility patients. Though it was wonderful to be caring for a couple from the egg retrieval to birth, the price was that my fertility patients inevitably paid for my hours in the delivery room. I couldn't be fully present for patients when I'd been up for forty-eight hours. I concluded it was best to follow my patients for the critical first twelve weeks of pregnancy, when almost all miscarriages occur, then send them to their regular ob/gyn.

The lessons I carried from Vancouver, of course, go far beyond those. Fertility treatment is a maelstrom for patients, an emotional and physiological whirlwind. I left Vancouver knowing how much patients need someone to step back and see their case from the nonemotional side, to synthesize their problem and come up with the essence of what they must do to go on. I left understanding how little power we truly have and how much responsibility.

Linda and Graham remain my close friends. They think that the extra two eggs Graham argued to transfer are the children they are raising.

As for the twelve-year-old twins, Mallory is deeply in love with horses. Every summer day she is at the barn. Taylor loves computers, Nintendo, and the Lord of the Rings. They fight like brothers and sisters do.

"Mom, he's hitting me," Mallory yells.

"No I'm not," Taylor shouts. "But I want to."

Sometimes, after a scary movie, Linda finds them in the same bed, curled together as they must have been in utero. They are tall and slender and trained in tae kwan do because Graham wants them to be survivors.

They don't know what survivors they are. How the boy blew a hole in his lung shortly after birth and scared us all. Or how, in the weeks after delivery, their mother was so weak from the bedrest that she would sit on the edge of the bed willing herself the strength to breast-feed. How she would sit next to the crib, hold the photograph of them just born in her hands, and cry for the miracle of it. They don't remember the trip to England when they were three to put flowers on their grandmother's grave. They don't remember. But their parents and I do, and have lived a bit differently ever since.

3 The Right Blend

They heard children everywhere they went in China. Shrieks of uniformed grade schoolers rose up from the schoolyard across the street from their hotel, catcalls from boys on bicycles, babies' cries in the market.

When the call came to their California home on a Saturday night in the spring of 1994, an adoption agent told Lynn and Tom that they had four days to get to China. The couple had been waiting for that call for nearly a year. Lynn landed in Shanghai Thursday at midnight, and by 6 A.M. she was en route to the orphanage. She had baby clothes, formula, disposable diapers, and the papers that had consumed most of their attention for the previous eight months. She had two months' leave from work and day care already lined up for when she eventually returned to the office. Lynn had considered everything. Except what lay ahead.

En route to the orphanage, the liaison told Lynn she was going to have to choose a baby.

"What?" she said. That wasn't how she wanted to build a family. Babies happened to you. Whether you adopted or gave birth, it was fate. You didn't choose, the universe did. God did. Her husband was half a world away traveling toward her. He wouldn't be there for another day. She would have to choose herself. Lynn knew by the time the orphanage doors opened that she would take the first child offered.

The infant, swaddled in thick, stiff cotton, was a wisp. Her black hair barely covered her tiny head. Her arms and legs were thin and wrinkled like an old man's, her belly protruded, her knees were sharp. She had no muscle tone. She was three and a half months old and weighed just over eight pounds. Her breathing was audible, like a whisper.

In the morning, Lynn had to take the baby girl to the hospital for the physical examination that would allow them to leave the country. Another American couple was waiting with their adopted baby. When they saw Lynn holding her infant, they blurted out that they had been shown her baby first. But they asked for another.

"We didn't think she was healthy enough," they said. "We didn't think she would live."

Years later, the memory of that statement could still choke Lynn to silence. She pulled her baby girl close.

When Tom arrived, they named her Elizabeth Quin. They flew home to their suburban life on the edge of the Silicon Valley. Lynn expected to be swept away by baby love. But she found that babies don't imprint like geese. The bond between a mother and child builds not in seconds, but in steps, repeated over months, individual acts of touch and cradle, bathe and feed. Until one morning she awoke and the bond was like iron.

I knew they had adopted a baby in China because Lynn and Tom had been pursuing in vitro fertilization with me at the same time.

The couple had met while working as computer programmers when they joined the same company in 1978. Tom taught Lynn to write her first program. Their relationship was in development longer than any product they ever worked on. After ten years of slow and easy friendship, Lynn realized there was something to be said for nice guys. She and Tom married. She was thirty-two. She'd grown up in San Francisco, the oldest of eight, and had left home at seventeen, in part to get away from the melee she had lived with there. One brother was autistic, and the responsibility and grief bore down on her parents so heavily that Lynn had no interest in becoming a parent. So her brothers and sisters were as shocked as she was when Lynn hit her mid-thirties and changed her mind. She had nieces and nephews practically in high school.

Sometimes you just grow into these things, she told the questioning clan. Tom reached the same point at about the same time, and they began trying to get pregnant around her thirty-fifth birthday. Lynn took her temperature every day before breakfast. Hormonal changes in the menstrual cycle affect a woman's body temperature, indicating if and when ovulation occurs. During the first two weeks of a cycle, a woman's temperature is relatively low. As the follicles on her ovaries develop, estrogen levels increase and then drop. This triggers a surge of the luteinizing hormone (LH), which converts the follicle from an estrogen-producing factory to a predominantly progesterone-producing factory. Progesterone raises the body temperature a half degree or more. Although temperature changes suggested Lynn was ovulating, she wasn't getting pregnant.

Lynn learned to check her cervical mucus, looking for the clear stretchy mucus resembling egg white that develops about two days before ovulation. She'd tell Tom it was time to have sex. She opened ovulation predictor kits, dipping a chemically prepared paper stick into her morning urine to monitor whether she had had the luteinizing hormone surge signaling that ovulation was imminent. If the paper stick changed color, they should be having what women in Internet chat rooms call "BMS"—baby-making sex. That night, the next night, and the next. She found herself actually saying, "We have to have sex *now*."

By thirty-seven Lynn had addressed every visible obstacle that might have been preventing pregnancy. Shortly before she came to me, she had laparoscopic surgery to straighten a kink in a fallopian tube and to remove some endometrial tissue, the result of endometriosis, a condition in which cells that are usually confined to the uterus, and that grow in response to estrogen, begin growing outside the uterus on the ovaries, bowel, and peritoneum, the membrane that covers all abdominal and pelvic organs.

I tell my patients that endometriosis can contribute to infertility either by causing a mechanical obstruction in the fallopian tubes or by causing lesions on the ovary. The condition can also trigger an abnormal immune response that interferes with fertilization and implantation of the embryo. Many women with endometriosis do get pregnant. But even mild endometriosis can decrease fertility by as much as one-third. Lynn had had her endometriosis treated with laser vaporization in her laparoscopic surgery several months earlier. The tissue can also be removed surgically or burned off with electrocauterization. But doctors are removing only the tissue they can see; there is some endometriosis that it is not possible to remove, and there is microscopic disease that doctors can't even see.

For years Lynn has had abdominal pain from endometriosis that seemed to peak in intensity between ovulation and her period. It doesn't surprise me that, by the time Lynn reaches our office, the pain has returned. The pain associated with endometriosis is unpredictable, and the severity of the symptoms may not be related to the extent of the disease. Some women with minimal disease have maximum pain and such symptoms as diarrhea, headache, abdominal pain, and cramps.

Lynn and Tom are pragmatists. In the months before they came to see me, they had agreed that they wanted at least two children. They thought they wouldn't be able to get pregnant twice through in vitro fertilization and so decided they would also pursue adoption in China.

The couple's adoption efforts were aided with some money Tom's parents had given the couple for a big family vacation. But when Tom and Lynn asked if they could put the money toward adoption instead, the prospective grandparents gave their warmest blessing. Tom and Lynn wanted a baby from China. That year it seems as if everyone did—a phenomenon that delayed their plans for parenthood.

Between 1992 and 1993, the number of Chinese babies being adopted by couples from the United States swelled. In response, the Chinese government temporarily put adoption applications on hold in order to revise its policies. As a result, Tom and Lynn's application went into a holding file for eight months. In those months of waiting for any news on China, Lynn and Tom decided to proceed with an in vitro fertilization cycle. They realized that the Chinese authorities might disapprove of a pregnant couple trying to adopt a child, so they agreed that if Lynn did get pregnant before their China adoption came through, Tom would go abroad alone.

We meet in my office on July 26, 1993. Lynn is thirty-eight. She has one ovary and fallopian tube on the left side. She lost her right fallopian tube and ovary when she was seventeen after an ovarian cyst ruptured. She told me that even with that loss, she never dreamed she'd have difficulty conceiving. But now the biological clock made the loss of that right ovary more acute. She had half the eggs she would have had otherwise, and age would soon compromise the ovary that remained. I had ordered blood tests that indicated Lynn's remaining ovary would be very hard to stimulate. She required the strongest regimen of fertility drugs.

But even with the most aggressive hormone prescriptions and two in vitro cycles, one in November 1993 and the other in March 1994, Lynn did not become pregnant. None of the transferred embryos implanted.

That's when, late that spring, Lynn and Tom went to China. They returned with little Elizabeth, who lights up their house with her growing, thriving self. Her tiny form quickly filled out and soon she grew into a gurgling, burping, and smiling baby. When Elizabeth was almost seven months old, Lynn and Tom stunned their friends and family by deciding to come back to my office in June 1994. The couple had paid for a plan that allows three in vitro cycles for $15,000. After two failed attempts, the couple figured that, if they were to have any chance of creating the family they'd dreamed of, they must act soon. I agreed. Friends and family are supportive to their faces, but in the years to come, these supporters will confess they were shocked and believed Lynn and Tom were "pushing their luck." But I could see how much they genuinely loved children. This couple wanted to extend their family, for themselves and for their daughter. When I asked how the little munchkin is, they spent several minutes describing Elizabeth's appetite and her latest milestone, which is sitting up on her own.

Looking at Lynn's previous cycles, I decide to back off the drug protocol a bit to see if, in her case, it might improve the egg quality. This time Lynn's single ovary produces four follicles, and we retrieve four eggs. Two fertilize with Tom's sperm and divide. But on the morning of the transfer, the embryologists in the laboratory inform me that both the embryos are heavily fragmented, that is, the cells are irregular in size and shape with dark bits or blemishes. Poorer-quality embryos don't make poorer-quality babies. But they do have less chance of successfully implanting. From where I sit, Lynn and Tom have about a 5 percent chance of becoming pregnant. It is a disappointment all around. We go into the transfer with a heavy heart.

After the transfer, Lynn is worried because she cannot lie down quietly for the following day or two, as many women do after the transfer. Unlike them, she has a seven-month-old infant at home to care for.

There is no hard science to support ordering someone to bed. Common sense tells us that most women should take it easy after the embryo transfer and should not exercise or overexert. But Lynn had a baby who needed her. How could I ask her not to lift a crying child? I try to ease her mind by telling her that most people who have sex and become pregnant spontaneously are not on strict bedrest around the time of implantation. I also tell her about a former patient who, based on a poor response, had only two embryos available for transfer. She was so discouraged that immediately after the procedure—and unbeknownst to me—she went home and went jogging. I learned of this after her pregnancy test was positive. Despite the run, she not only conceived, she delivered a healthy child.

Nevertheless, Lynn leaves my office as that patient did—assuming the cycle failed. When our staff nurse calls to remind her to come in for the pregnancy test a week later, Lynn protests that she doesn't see the point. Finally, she relents and comes in.

The test is positive. Lynn cannot believe it. She had such a slim shot at success that it cannot be true. But the pregnancy hormone levels in her blood keep rising. "It's more than a nibble," I tell her. Finally, at six weeks, when I'm able to point out the fluttering pulse of a heartbeat on the ultrasound monitor, Lynn and Tom become very excited. These moments are the ones that are so fulfilling to share with my patients.

Several weeks later, Lynn is driving home after work when her 1984 Honda quits on Interstate 880. She walks three miles to the nearest exit. No one stops; even a police car passes her without slowing. By the time she reaches a gas station and calls home, she is overheated, furious, and frightened. She is bleeding. She calls me, panicked. I reassure her and arrange for her to come to the office the next morning for an ultrasound to check the baby.

The baby is fine, but I certainly understand why Lynn was so worried. The sight of blood is always alarming for an expectant mother. Up to 20 percent of women will have some sort of spotting in the first trimester, I tell her. Sometimes it comes from the implantation site or an irritation of the cervix. In rare cases, a woman may continue to bleed at the expected time of her period throughout the first or even second trimester. For reasons I really can't explain, Lynn has placental bleeding that continues throughout the entire pregnancy. The blood makes Lynn so nervous that she wants to buy a Doppler device so she can constantly monitor the baby's heartbeat between appointments. Her pregnancy is, in other respects, textbook healthy, but Lynn enjoys none of it. The bleeding is a constant worry. She tells few people about the baby; she is afraid she'll somehow jinx it. Most people don't even realize she and Tom are expecting until she is an unmistakable eight months along.

A week before her fortieth birthday, Lynn goes into labor. All her life she has expected labor to be a noisy, violent experience. But her labor and delivery are so efficient and relaxed that the hospital turns Tom's birth video into its Lamaze training film. Their baby is a girl, Rebecca, eight pounds, eight ounces. Lynn feels the same curious connection she did with Elizabeth. Not an instant bonding at all, but a long, slow slide into love. Their two daughters grow beautifully, one black-haired with dark eyes, one blonde with dark eyes. Lynn and Tom love the noise and joys of parenthood. Lynn tells people that, if she wins the lottery, she would use it for another in vitro or adoption attempt. She wants to try to have even more children—"a whole bunch." Tom is a "Thomas II" and he'd have liked a "Thomas III." He wants a boy to carry on the family name and to give his father a grandson.

It all seems like a pipe dream until the couple has a windfall. They don't win the lottery, but when Lynn's company is sold, she receives an eight-month severance package. The couple immediately goes down to the car dealership to look for a new truck. As they stand next to each other reading the $26,000 price sticker, they decide they'd rather have their family grow than have a four-wheel drive. That's when they called on me again.

It's like a reunion. When Lynn and Tom come into my office, I push my chair back and start talking. Having them return to discuss having another child just affirms for me what a good experience parenthood has been for them. It's gratifying to see people who truly are happy with the outcome. Lynn has photos of the daughter we helped them have, Rebecca, and their daughter from China, Elizabeth Quin. Lynn's great-grandfather was from China. My wife, Miriam, was also born in China.

Miriam's family immigrated to Canada when she was a child. When Miriam, as a Canadian doctor on holiday, visited her native village years later, she realized that, had she remained in China, her whole world would have been her village and perhaps the one next to it. She vividly remembers at age three standing in line with many sick people waiting all day to see a doctor. She decided then to become a doctor herself, and when her family immigrated to Canada, she did just that. Miriam says that her family's struggle to escape communism opened the door to her good fortune. She tells me that among the Chinese characters that form the word *crisis* is the character for the word *opportunity*.

Lynn and Tom's struggle with infertility opened the door to their daughter Elizabeth's good fortune. I can see in the photos that the underweight, orphaned baby has become a sturdy, secure, and beautiful little girl. Her parents tell me they want to give the girls another sibling. But, with Lynn nearing forty-two, and their previous experience, the chances of their becoming pregnant again with her own eggs are slim. I tell them they need to consider an egg donor.

Egg donation was first suggested to help women with premature ovarian failure. But it quickly became a way for mature women facing the natural decline in fertility to extend their ability to become pregnant, deliver, and nurture a baby. As long as a woman is healthy, her ability to carry a baby does not decline with age, but her ability to conceive with her own eggs does. The most important predictor of success is the age of the egg.

Lynn isn't worried about raising a child that isn't genetically hers. Raising Elizabeth and Rebecca has convinced her that a family is more than a gene pool. She and Tom want the best chance to take home a baby, and a young donor with young eggs offers that chance.

The use of genetically unrelated donor eggs is one of the areas in which reproductive medicine is changing the way people build families. But it doesn't change what a family is. "The basis of a family is love and support and not genetic inheritance," says the ethicist David Thomasma. That some children in Lynn and Tom's family will be genetically linked to their parents and others will not is neither radical nor extreme. Complex family relationships already exist in our world—they have since medieval kings married the wives of their dead brothers. And they certainly exist without assisted reproduction. We all know families with multiple marriages that combine children from each previous union. Throughout history, humans have proven remarkably capable of adapting to disruptions and disjunctions in the family fabric. While we may be giving Lynn and Tom a new way to extend their family, we are not changing what the essence of their family will be.

Lynn and Tom are open to the idea of using an anonymous egg donor, but they wonder how they can afford it. Looking at the figures, they realize the cost would swallow what they have saved to buy a family home in a good public school district.

They then learn of the shared-ovum donor program. Under the program, two couples separately and anonymously select the same egg donor. She is stimulated with fertility drugs, and her eggs are retrieved. The eggs are then divided between the two recipients. The eggs are fertilized by the respective fathers and then transferred into the intended mothers, just as in any in vitro fertilization cycle. The two couples never meet. Their appointments are deliberately scheduled at different times to avoid an accidental meeting. The program is anonymous—no names, addresses, or phone numbers are ever exchanged. But both couples have the option of sending a letter to the donor through the center. Some families have no contact with their egg donor, but others write thank-you notes and even send flowers.

By California law, the eggs and the resulting embryos are treated as property and thus bound by the same statutes that govern property issues.

The logistics of sharing an egg donor—of preparing all the parties, timing the cycles of three women, and completing the necessary legal agreements beforehand—are among the most complicated in in vitro fertilization. But the cost is about half that of using an egg donor exclusively, because the two couples share the cost of the donor's evaluation, treatment, and compensation. For someone like Lynn, whose resistant ovaries will need very costly amounts of fertility drugs to complete a cycle, the shared program can be even less expensive than if she were to use her own eggs. One downside may be that, if a couple doesn't conceive, they are less likely to have frozen embryos remaining for another try.

Lynn and Tom make an appointment at the agency and sit next to each other looking through big black three-ring binders for a potential match. It's a strange feeling to be looking at photos and medical histories of the potential genetic mother of their child. They have agreed on certain criteria.

Tom is a cup right out of the melting pot: His ancestors were German, English, Scottish, and Native American. Lynn's ancestry is even more diverse and included South American Indian, African American, Chinese, and northern European. Because of Lynn's heritage and their adopted daughter, they'd like to use an Asian egg donor. An Amerasian child seems the right blend between Elizabeth and Rebecca, a reflection of their unique family. Lynn and Tom are people of medium height. They'd like a donor who is at least five feet, seven inches, because to them it seems the world gives tall people a better shake. They'd prefer someone who looks a little like Lynn, who is in excellent health, and, since they both wear glasses, someone who has good eyes.

The Asian donors available, though, are of Pacific Island descent, not Chinese. No one looks like Lynn. After a fruitless search, Lynn concludes she doesn't care as long as the donor isn't short.

The egg donor they choose is five feet, two inches. She is blond, twenty-five, and has two children of her own. She has donated twice before, and each time the couple took home a baby. She writes that if she could pass on a message with her eggs, it is, "Enjoy every moment of parenthood and give your child all the love you can." That she is short suddenly doesn't matter at all. She is healthy and gorgeous and strikes them as being the absolute right blend. Another couple agrees and chooses her, too. In December, the three women, all strangers to one another, complete all psychological and medical tests and begin taking birth control pills to synchronize their cycles.

The donor's eggs are retrieved late in January. She produces twenty-six eggs. Tom and Lynn get thirteen. In the laboratory, twelve of the eggs fertilize with Tom's sperm, and, by the morning of the transfer, eight are graded as very good to excellent. Lynn and Tom can't believe it. At the pretransfer conference on January 25, we discuss how many embryos to put back. In their previous cycles, only one of the twelve embryos we transferred into Lynn implanted. This time, though, we're using young donor eggs. Transferring more embryos does increase the likelihood that she'll become pregnant. Here is our dilemma: On the one hand, this couple cannot afford to do this again. On the other hand, the more aggressive we are, the higher the chance of a major multiple pregnancy.

If a couple can consider selective reduction to protect the health of the mother and the future children in the event that more than two implant, we can be more aggressive with the transfer. If a selective reduction is not an acceptable alternative for religious, moral, or ethical reasons, then we must back off on the number of embryos we transfer, knowing that this approach also reduces the chances of our winding up with a baby. Within eighteen months of this conversation, we'll have the option of transferring just one embryo with the same success. By that time our center will have a new culture medium that will allow us to grow the embryos longer in the laboratory and thus transfer embryos in the blastocyst stage or more robust stage. But as Lynn and Tom and I talk, that new culture medium is still at least a year away. At this point in time, Lynn and Tom and I must discuss the risk of a major multiple. Lynn and Tom say they can reduce, knowing there is no way she could carry three or more babies. On the basis of her history of problems with implantation, we decide to transfer five. Ten days after the transfer, tests indicate Lynn is pregnant, and the pregnancy hormones in her blood are rising at a rate that can only mean she's pregnant with more than one baby. Lynn is calm, though; she stays busy at work and home and believes that nature will take care of what comes next. She trusts the process. This time the ultrasound at six weeks shows there are three separate sacs with very clear fetal heartbeats. All these years with barely a nibble, and now she has three.

I tell her that there is almost a 20 percent chance that one of the three will be reabsorbed between the sixth and tenth week. Nature seems to conduct quality control during these weeks, and it is not unusual for one of those early sacs to disappear. We call it the vanishing twin. Lynn is soon bleeding again, and she is convinced that one of three sacs is being reabsorbed. But an ultrasound at eight weeks in March shows that all three sacs are present with heartbeats. For a moment, Lynn, Tom, and I watch the ultrasound monitor, silent. For me, this is not a success. To have three fetuses at the end of eight or nine weeks is more than we wanted. What strikes me most is the enormity of the decision that comes next. And the guilt and anguish that will accompany Lynn and Tom as they face it. We have to consider terminating one of the apparently healthy fetuses.

From a strictly medical point of view, carrying more than two babies increases the risks to Lynn's health and to the health of her unborn babies. Lynn's pregnancy is already high-risk. She could lose the entire pregnancy.

Intellectually Lynn understood our discussion in the pretransfer conference, and my concern about the risk to herself and the babies if the pregnancy continues. She has heard about the dangers and long-term effects of premature birth. But emotionally, she says she feels like she's in a funnel with no exit, trapped by the potentially devastating pregnancy and birth, by the image of trying to raise five children, and by the decision she and Tom must make. She is a mother, she has responsibility to her other children and to the potential children she carries. What she knows she must do fills her, at this most expectant time, with the deepest grief.

They have the reduction. An ultrasound in the weeks after confirms a healthy ongoing pregnancy. The two fetuses are growing, the tiny third sac still visible but shrinking. Lynn is relieved when the other two get big enough on the ultrasound monitor to blot it out.

Several weeks later Tom's father, Thomas, dies. He was a loving, inspirational man, and they are knocked backward by his sudden death. They undergo amniocentesis at sixteen weeks so they can learn the sex of the twins for his mother. They announce it at the funeral. A girl and a boy.

Postscript

Six and a half months into the pregnancy, Tom was in Alaska wrapping up property issues from his father's estate when Lynn, who was working and caring for the girls, started bleeding. The doctor ruled out placenta previa and during an internal examination found she was 100 percent effaced, her cervix thinned completely in preparation for labor. She was about to deliver the babies fourteen weeks early.

She was admitted to the hospital and given medications that relax the uterus to try to stave off labor for another two weeks. When the medication ceased to be effective, a delivery was planned. But one of the placentas had begun to separate from the uterine wall, causing massive internal hemorrhaging. Lynn was rushed in for an emergency cesarean section.

The twins were born weighing three pounds, nine ounces and two pounds, ten ounces. The biggest, the boy, was silent. He was whisked away before his mother could see him. She had only the briefest glimpse of their girl. Lynn had lost a lot of blood and was shaky and weak after her surgery. But the babies were in far worse shape.

Thomas III was bleeding in his brain. The size of his head was growing from the accumulated fluid. The next morning the doctor said they needed to consider removing life support. And if the baby survived, he likely faced major disabilities. Doctors also discovered that one of his heart valves had remained open, shunting blood away from his lungs. As a result, his skin color was a distinct purplish blue. His twin, Tara, had her own struggle with a blood infection, and she required several blood transfusions.

Had the twins come any earlier, or been a fraction smaller, they might never have survived, the staff told Lynn. But the twins were survivors. Within two weeks, miraculously, the bleeding in Thomas III's brain was no longer detectable, and his heart problem was repaired with medication. Tom began bringing the girls to the hospital to see their brother and sister. Thomas III and Tara spent a total of seventy-two and ninety-two days, respectively, in the hospital. Their mother came every day with breast milk; she got up every morning at 4:30 A.M. to pump her milk so they would have enough. Her schedule was almost inhumanely exhausting, but Lynn was determined to give the twins all the help she and Tom could. When they were released from the hospital, the infants were on baby monitors and oxygen for several months. The household was thrown into constant chaos day and night by alarms going off. This continued until the twins reached eight months.

At eleven months, Lynn and Tom finally made a conscious decision to let the babies cry themselves to sleep. It was time to begin to treat them normally. They were crawling and cruising, like any nine month olds, their corrected age. Miraculously, Thomas has met every developmental milestone.

Sometimes, the family watches the video of the orphanage in China. They watch the training film on Rebecca's letter-perfect birth. The older girls are so close that Rebecca's heart was broken when her big sister started school. They have each other; the twins have each other; and Lynn and Tom have each other. "It's nice to be part of a pair," Lynn says.

Lynn thinks sometimes about the egg donor who helped them. She wishes there was a centralized donor registry collecting information on the outcome of egg and sperm donation. Their donor has two children of her own and has helped other families, and Lynn and Tom would like information on any half-siblings.

They recently finished a letter to the egg donor, thanking her for what she gave them. They plan to send it with a gift, a porcelain figurine of a mother and child that says "A mother's love is forever." The child represents the donor's children and their children. Lynn keeps meaning to send it. But their lives are busy and messy and full of love, which seems to Lynn the absolute right blend.

4 Hope

*I*n the ten years before I came to San Francisco, my practice in Vancouver included helping infertile couples to conceive and supervising high-risk pregnancies through to safe delivery. I have held many, many babies who made it against all odds and some babies who didn't. I have stood in operating rooms in the middle of the night, drawing on hidden reserves of medical expertise, adrenaline, and prayer.

Most of obstetrics goes as smoothly as we can hope and as nature intends. Perhaps one in every ten cases is a challenging, but manageable, labor and delivery. One in every twenty, though, has the potential to go from problematic to absolute blind terror, with the mother having seizures, uncontrollable hemorrhaging, or a catastrophic system failure. You come out of such experiences humbled by the mysteries of the human body, the intuition of pregnant women, and the spirit it takes to be alive.

I see that spirit, that mystery, and often, that loss, each day in the lives of my patients. Many of the couples come to me from the bereavement of miscarriage or stillbirth. Other patients have had older children who died accidentally or from disease. A letter arrives on my desk with news that a family I had helped had lost their baby at two months of age to sudden infant death syndrome. I pick up the telephone to call the couple immediately, and all I can say when the mother answers is that I'm sorry, it is just so unfair. All I can really do is listen.

When a child dies, the grief seeps far beyond the immediate loss. It is the loss of the present and the loss of the future. You cannot replace that child, ever. You cannot replace one individual with a new one, like you get a new car after an accident. Yet the birth of other children, as separate and unique individuals, as gifts in their own right, is what we hope for. It's part of the renewal of life that keeps me in this field and gives me personal hope for the patients who've dealt with death.

In fertility medicine, as in life, there are losses other than death. There is the loss of the prospect of a perfect child, the child we all dreamed of one day having. For some, that is the loss of a daughter when the baby turns out to be a son, or vice versa. For other couples, who have twins or triplets because of fertility treatment, it is the loss of a "normal" family with years of spacing between the children. For infertile couples who need donated eggs or sperm to conceive, there is the loss of having one's own genetic child. There is the loss that becomes the endpoint for couples who choose to stop treatment and live child-free. These are quiet surrenders that leave lifelong marks. They have taught me much about loss, and my experience as a husband and father has shaped me as well.

I met my wife, Miriam Jang, through another couple's struggle with infertility. In the late 1980s, Miriam was a family doctor in Vancouver, British Columbia, and had privileges at the same hospital that I did, but we didn't know each other. When one of Miriam's friends had difficulty conceiving, Miriam made the referral that eventually brought the friend to me. The friend became pregnant and delivered a child, then invited both Miriam and me to the celebratory baby banquet with the intention of introducing us.

Miriam came to the party with a girlfriend, expecting the introduction to take place. Oblivious to this plan, I came with a date. Miriam was so put off that she claims she glared at me during hospital staff meetings for the next two years. Then I was seated next to her at the hospital Christmas party. We talked the entire evening. Within three months, we were engaged; three months after that, we were married. We had different backgrounds and yet shared these same beliefs: a common desire to help others, to make a difference in the world, and at the same time, to grow spiritually.

My patients sometimes ask what religion I am, and I tell them that we celebrate every holiday at our home. My grandparents were Greek Orthodox, but there were no Greek Orthodox churches in the South African city where I was raised, so I was brought up in the Anglican church. I was educated by the Christian Brothers, who were mostly Irish, in a parochial school. After my brother and father died, my mother in her grief sought and found solace in yoga and the principles of Hinduism. Miriam was influenced by both Eastern religions and Christianity. I meditate as often as I can, as soon as I get up in the morning, and I have borrowed a little from every major religion that has touched my life. Miriam and I both believe that the basis of our spiritual life is the willingness or call to help others. We were well into our thirties when we met and had a wide range of life and professional experiences, yet it was the simplest thing that seems to have changed us and deepened our faith profoundly. We became parents.

When our daughter, Natasha, was born, our world changed. I thought that, because I had delivered nearly two thousand babies and worked with so many couples with infertility problems, I understood the miracle of birth. But when Natasha was born, it was as if for years I'd been listening to music in monotone and suddenly I was standing in front of the whole orchestra. The wonder was magnified a thousand times. Miriam said that she never saw herself as the maternal type, but when she became a mom she developed an appreciation for all children. Dr. Jang was suddenly asking to hold patients' babies or coming out to the waiting room to see a child. Concerns or worries that Miriam and I used to dismiss as overprotectiveness on the part of our patients suddenly made perfect sense. When Miriam took Natasha in for an immunization shot, she worried that our baby might catch a cold from the sick toddler also in the pediatrician's waiting room. I couldn't believe the tender feelings this baby awakened. When my wife and daughter came home from the hospital, we borrowed an acrylic bassinet from the nursery just so we could watch Natasha sleep.

When Natasha was almost two years old, we were fortunate enough to have a son, Marc, every bit the miracle and so like his sister in looks. I videotaped little Marky's birth, as I had Natasha's. We felt we had the family we had prayed for, with whispered thanks that we had escaped the anguish that every one of my patients faced. It was uncommon luck. Within the year, I took the position in San Francisco. It was a massive move, as Miriam and I had both lived and practiced medicine in Canada for most of our adult lives. Despite the move, we expected life would continue pretty much as it always had: busy and divided between caring for our patients and our children.

I remember the first time we looked at each other and knew that something was wrong. Marky was two and a half years old when he just stopped talking. He stopped looking at us. He refused any food except Chee•tos and soy milk. One day Miriam found him in a closet, wedged tightly between some boxes and the wall. Other days he seemed to want to sleep under the mattress. He threw confounding tantrums. We lay awake at night and talked and talked about his behavior. Looking back now, it is so easy to see the signs. But at the time, Miriam and I followed the advice that we had given numerous patients who were worried about their kids: Don't compare your children; it's just a phase; it will pass.

It was not just a phase. When we enrolled Marky in nursery school, the teacher asked us if he was deaf. He doesn't pay attention, she said. Eventually, like a hole widening in a dam, the diagnosis was made. Marky has autism, a term that describes a range of neurologic disorders that affect language, social skills, sensory contact, and abstract thought. Sights, sounds, touches, and tastes can overwhelm the child. In autism, children are basically in their own world until they can be enticed back to our world.

I don't think Miriam and I ate a normal meal or slept a normal night for the next three years. We wanted to deny it, but we couldn't afford the luxury of denial. We knew that the earlier we intervened with therapy, the better chance there was that Marky's neuropathways would develop. We knew that Marky would never be three years old again. So Miriam quit the family practice she loved and for which she was beloved. With tutors, she began working with Marky eight hours a day, seven days a week. We followed the principles of Lovaas, a behavior modification program, developed by Dr. Ivar Lovaas at UCLA, that attempts to imprint verbal and social skills, to help the auditory processing, as well as to stimulate physical movement and balance in autistic children like Marky. You basically break a task down into its most basic elements and repeat those actions over and over. Miriam and the tutors worked and worked, sometimes saying the same word to Marky two thousand times.

The first year he learned so much. The second year he lost all of it. I was crushed. Miriam was in such despair that the normal joys of life for her disappeared. Natasha would say, "Mommy and Daddy, you're not listening." We were distracted, consumed with the next step. Time or grace or God seemed to mobilize us to try again. Miriam says I'm a rock, but she's the one who kept our family going, who still keeps us going, searching and trying therapies. She recently became trained in OPTIONS, a form of therapy that uses play and validation of a child's behavior to draw him out emotionally.

I don't talk to most of my patients about Marky's autism. I may say something to a special education teacher whom I'm treating, or perhaps to a couple who also has a disabled child. When I once told a reporter, she said that she thought I was trying to win her sympathy with the information.

I don't intentionally bring autism to work, but it follows me anyway. I hear my patients describe their painful quest to have a family, and they could be describing our search for a cure. It's an exact mirror process. Even the diagnosis brings about the same reactions: First the question Why me? then feelings of anger, depression, and finally resolve. With Marky, a cold or a trip can cause a complete regression, and it's like getting a positive pregnancy test that disappears. It knocks you down.

When Miriam was younger, she prayed for spiritual growth, which, for her, meant compassion, humility, and patience. Autism and infertility evoke all of those. You are humbled because, in every other aspect of life, when you want something, you work for it and it happens. In autism and infertility, you can push and push without any progress. If you just knew the answer, you would follow any protocol. But you don't know. You are not in control.

Patients talk about infertility changing every aspect of their lives and I understand. For years, we have avoided situations that might be uncomfortable, like attending birthday parties or visiting with Santa— the kind of outings that can overwhelm Marky's senses. We found ourselves avoiding other families, even those with autistic children, because comparisons are inevitable and often depressing. The smallest things separate you from everyone else. My wife and I were at a friend's wedding recently, feeling joy for the couple and, at the same time, such sadness that our son may never marry.

One of my fondest memories is of Natasha as a toddler following me in and out of the garage as I was building our backyard fence, asking questions, carrying tools, being such a little helper. Natasha's curiosity, her ability to extrapolate and integrate new knowledge into her existing body of knowledge, her artistic and musical creativity and empathy for others astonished and delighted us. We were grateful for her gifts. But we took them for granted. Who knew that one day we would be grateful just to have our son be able to say a word, any word, or show normal interest in a toy. It's like the couples who take it for granted that they'll become pregnant when they want, never realizing that for others getting pregnant will take a miracle. The trick is truly to appreciate the everyday miracles and the things that go right before we get the wake-up call. Perhaps that is what enlightenment is.

Miriam and I have learned from our son who could not communicate to appreciate the amazing process of learning and the acquisition of language. At the mall, when I hear parents tell their kids, "Shut up" or "Don't ask so many questions," it's like a dagger to the heart. People are always telling my patients that suffering makes you stronger. They tell my wife the same thing. But I think suffering makes you softer, makes your compassion grow, and creates within you a tenderness toward the world, a reverence for the gifts we walk by daily. You never again take it for granted when a child blurts something out or picks up a toy car and plays with it appropriately. These are hard-won graces.

Shortly after Marky's diagnosis, a specialist told my wife that there was no hope for him and that he would never talk. The pain in Miriam's face when she told me this deepened my resolve not ever to do that to my patients. There is hope, always hope, only hope. When Marky was diagnosed, there was almost no bond between the two of us. Today he asks me for a Coke or milk and gives me "high fives" and kisses. He loves it at night when I cuddle him and Natasha, who teases me for always falling asleep as she reads their bedtime story. When Marky smiles at me with that little toothy grin, it is the most beautiful sight in the world, because an autistic child is incapable of artifice or superficiality. Marky's smile is pure. I see my wife in the doorway watching us, and the smile on her face is pure, too. This image I carry to my practice and my patients: No one in the world, not the highest or best-trained specialist, has the right to take away a family's hope.

5 The Rigors of the Science

Cheryl lived most things twice. She tended to worry about circumstances in her life before they happened. Often this led her to envision an event in advance, and then to live it again in real time. She worried about her two children and their health and their grades; she worried about her husband, Rick, and his new company; she worried about her old company, a department store that folded. She worried about her age. She was like an antenna that her husband teasingly said was always tuned to the worst. But infertility medicine was like nothing she'd ever encountered.

When Cheryl met Rick, she was a thirty-four-year-old divorced mother of two; he was thirty and had not been married before. They married in 1994 and started trying to have a baby the following spring. Cheryl wanted to have another child, and she wanted Rick to experience all the wonders she had parenting. They came to the marriage matured from three decades of life, but their relationship was like new love, full of hope and aspiration and a desire to have a family and a life together.

Cheryl had conceived so easily with her older children that, when she didn't conceive after six months of trying with Rick, they went in for testing. X rays showed that her tubes were clear and that she was ovulating, but Rick's sperm count was low. The doctor recommended artificial insemination. They tried six times. As the months passed, Cheryl's hopes would rise. Then her period would start, and they would plummet. Seeing other women with babies brought a lump to her throat. Cheryl started feeling as though everyone could conceive but her. She became increasingly concerned that time would run out for Rick and her.

When their doctor advised them to consider in vitro fertilization, all roads seemed to lead to our center. A friend of a friend had gotten pregnant there, and Rick had just seen an article in *The New York Times* on the shared risk program. As they made an appointment, her biggest worry was that she'd have to do more than one cycle.

Even at the point the staff was explaining the regimen of shots, Cheryl didn't quite realize all the problems she would need to address. No way did she think she would wind up having more than 250 injections. She could not imagine heparin shots to the stomach twice a day. And she certainly never saw herself as an unusual case.

When I meet Cheryl and Rick, she is thirty-nine, and he is thirty-five, and we need to figure out what we're up against. For Cheryl, and for all the patients who arrive at my office, careful preliminary testing is the first and critical step in an in vitro fertilization cycle. I need the information those tests provide to identify the variables in each person's case and to learn which ones the couple and I can change. On the first or second trip to the center, a woman must have ten to twelve test tubes of blood drawn. It is daunting but necessary. The tests give us the road map for the journey to come.

First, I order a blood test on the second or third day of a woman's menstrual cycle to measure the level of follicle-stimulating hormone (FSH) and estradiol. These numbers tell me how each patient will likely respond to fertility drugs. They help me gauge the right amount of medication to prescribe. For instance, a woman who is close to the end of her supply of eggs has a higher level of FSH as the pituitary gland struggles to push the ovaries to respond. Ideally, the FSH should be lower than 10 mIU/ml and the level of estradiol should be less than 70 pg/ml.

As the ovarian follicles grow, they produce more and more estrogen. The level of Cheryl's estradiol becomes the yardstick that I use when I chart the progress of the follicles. By monitoring the amount of estradiol in the blood, I can determine how the ovaries are responding to the fertility drugs. These results allow me to adjust the dose and duration of the fertility medication to get the best results and avoid any serious side effects.

Blood is also drawn to test for infectious diseases in both partners and also for immunity to rubella. A basic immune panel includes tests for thyroid antibodies, antibodies to sperm, and the full panel of antiphospholipid antibodies. Where there is evidence of previous pregnancy loss or repeat failed IVF attempts, the immunological testing will be more extensive and include testing for the presence of a natural killer (NK) cell, antipaternal leukocyte antibodies, and the DQ alpha genotype of both partners.

I believe that the immune system may be responsible for failed IVF and pregnancy loss in the following ways: Some women produce autoantibodies that attack the membranes of the cells that surround the developing embryo, the cells destined to become the early placenta. These antibodies, known as antiphospholipid antibodies, attack the cells of the implanting embryo's root system and can cause blood clots in the small blood vessels of the developing placenta. A woman may also produce antithyroid antibodies that can inhibit the differentiation of the cytotrophoblast, which is the mass of cells that is the early embryo, into the syncytiotrophoblast, which is the second line of cells to develop and the trigger that produces hormones including the pregnancy hormone, human chorionic gonadotrophin (hCG). The thyroid antibody can prevent the differentiation so that some women with thyroid antibodies may have early implantation but experience negative pregnancy tests. We also need to consider that a woman's body may fail to produce certain alloantibodies, the protective blocking antibodies needed to keep her immune system from rejecting the embryos as a foreign tissue. The third component of the immune system, the cells, in the form of natural killer cells, needs to be checked to exclude any situation in which these usually protective lymphocytes are directed to attack the pregnancy. Normally, these white blood cells function as the body's defense and attack invaders like viruses, bacteria, and tumor cells. In some women, these cells become misdirected and fail to distinguish between a tumor and an embryo.

Each human being has a certain unique genetic makeup to his or her tissues. In the DQ alpha genotype test, we look at two specific markers that are very similar to the bar codes that are printed on goods in a supermarket. When the clerk runs the product across the laser scanner, the central computer is able to tell a lot about that product. The bar code is an identifier to the central computer about the nature of that product. In the same way, every human being has, in the DQ alpha system, two "bar codes"; these transmit certain genetic information to the immune system. If a couple shares the same DQ alpha bar codes, or if one or both of them have a number 4 as one of their bar codes, the resulting embryos may have a tougher time implanting and remaining implanted because they may elicit an attack response from the mother instead of a protective response.

After these blood tests are complete, I perform the physical examinations, including taking cervical cultures for sexually transmitted diseases and doing a hysteroscopy, which allows me directly to examine the uterus. During the hysteroscopy, I pass a thin telescope-like instrument through the vagina, through the cervix, and into the uterus. This is usually done under light anesthetic, and carbon dioxide is used to inflate the uterus slightly so I can better see it in its entirety.

We're equal opportunity testers, I tell Cheryl. Rick will also be tested for ureaplasma, chlamydia, gonorrhea, and routine bacteria, as well as HIV, sperm antibodies, and a semen analysis. It generally takes four to six weeks to complete these tests and costs about $3,000 for both parties. Insurance often covers these diagnostic procedures. Many patients do all the testing beforehand with their own physician before coming to me for treatment.

In Rick and Cheryl's case, they finish the testing, and I review the results. The tests show that Rick's sperm count, which was low enough to prompt the six insemination attempts, is normal now. Cheryl already has had two children; she's had ovarian cysts and mild endometriosis diagnosed in the past. Endometriosis is a condition that can trigger an immune response. Indeed, she tests positive for antiphospholipid antibodies, which attack the cells that hold together the early embryo and early placenta. To help her conceive, I determine Cheryl needs immunotherapy, including heparin and aspirin.

Now I also have to pick the right fertility drug protocol for Cheryl. I suspect she will be a high responder, on the basis of her menstrual history. When a woman has a cycle longer than twenty-eight or twenty-nine days, I can predict she will likely be very responsive and make more than the average number of follicles for her age. Cheryl's period occurs every thirty-one to thirty-two days. But the follicle-stimulating hormone levels in Cheryl's blood tested on the third day of her cycle contradict this supposition. The FSH level is high, indicating that her ovaries may be starting to gradually decrease their production of eggs. So, on the one hand, her menstrual history predicts that she's going to respond well to ovulation drugs, and on the other hand, her FSH level is telling us she may be moderately resistant. The level of follicle-stimulating hormone is nine, which is very close to the ten that predicts resistance. I'm on the horns of a dilemma here. Cheryl has never taken fertility drugs. If I'm not aggressive, she may not get many follicles. But if she's a high responder, and I give her an aggressive protocol, she'll be at risk for hyperstimulation.

Severe ovarian hyperstimulation syndrome (OHSS) is the most common and, in very rare cases, deadly complication of fertility drugs. Whenever a woman makes more than twenty follicles and her estrogen levels rise to more than 6,000 picograms per milliliter, there is nearly an 80 percent chance of severe hyperstimulation syndrome developing. When it occurs, the ovaries become enlarged and tender. Fluid—mostly water with various mixture of protein and electrolytes—accumulates in the abdomen as the follicles grow. Once an hCG shot is given to trigger maturation of the eggs, the symptoms gradually worsen, then peak about a week later. But if the patient gets pregnant, the symptoms and risks may persist for nine weeks. In the worse cases, massive amounts of fluid, which the body cannot flush out as urine, accumulate in the abdomen, thereby compromising kidney function. At this point, I must sometimes go in and remove some of the fluid to relieve the pressure. I do this using the same technique that I use for an egg retrieval: pushing an aspiration needle through the vaginal wall to reach the fluid behind the uterus. In the worst cases, as much as three to five liters of fluid may be drawn off. This is a rare occurrence, happening perhaps in only four cases out of a thousand a year in our clinic. Blood tests help me monitor a woman's risk for OHSS and to respond immediately.

National statistics show the risk of moderate and severe hyperstimulation is about 3 to 4 percent. Many clinics cancel the cycle at the first sign of hyperstimulation. The staff calls off the egg retrieval and sends the patient home. The eggs are reabsorbed by the body. I imagine what it feels like to be that patient, the time and money she has invested are gone. The follicles that she watched grow and their cargo, the eggs, are lost. The patient is told she's responded too well.

There's no need to cancel cycles because of the fear of severe ovarian hyperstimulation syndrome. In 1993, my partners and I first described "prolonged coasting," which is a technique that allows us to continue the cycle without the risk of life-threatening consequences. Coasting works like this: Any patient with more than twenty follicles after a week on fertility drugs is at risk if her estradiol level is projected to rise over 3,000 picograms per milliliter. Once the follicles reach 15 to 16 millimeters in size, additional fertility drugs are withheld. The patient continues the drug Lupron so ovulation doesn't inadvertently take place. Gradually, the estradiol produced by the follicles drops to a safe level of 3,000 pg/ml. At that point, we can order the shot of hCG to trigger the final egg maturation, and proceed with the cycle. The eggs are retrieved; the patient is safe; and we have a good yield of mature eggs.

Why do we want Cheryl to make so many eggs? Because the only way you can twist nature's arm and defy the biological clock is to have a large pool of embryos. At thirty-nine and beyond, the more embryos a couple produces, the more likely she and her partner are to have ones that are chromosomally normal and, thus, more likely to implant and grow into a healthy baby. Knowing that we can coast, I decide to stimulate Cheryl as if she may not respond well. Based on her age and FSH level, I choose the strongest protocol.

As my staff and I discuss the treatment with her, I see that Cheryl is getting very nervous about all the shots and medication. Looking at her calendar printed up by her clinical coordinator, she suddenly confronts the prospect of as many as nineteen birth control pills and twenty-one shots of Lupron to suppress her own hormonal system. The medication will put her in a temporary menopausal state so that, when she begins taking fertility drugs, she will not have an inopportune ovulation. Next will come an injection of a fertility drug once a day for at least eight days and two shots of heparin a day for eight days. In other words, she'll be getting fifty-five shots before she even gets to the embryo transfer.

If she becomes pregnant, she'll have about seventy shots of progesterone and twice daily shots of heparin for twelve weeks, for a total of 238 shots after the transfer. Now, in 1999, progesterone is taken both vaginally and orally at the same time, a development that makes the luteal phase support for all assisted reproductive cycles nearly injection-free. But this development is still two years away for Cheryl. She'll have to have all of these shots.

When Cheryl realizes the extent of the injections, Rick is out of town on business for his small technology marketing company. Cheryl is practically screaming, "Let's just forget this whole thing." She is stopped by a small nagging internal voice. What if she doesn't do it? She will always wonder what might have been. She calls a friend who is a nurse and who agrees to help her start the shots. Rick takes over the injections when he returns home.

Rick carefully injected Lupron into the fatty portion of Cheryl's upper thigh with a short, thin needle. After she has received ten days of Lupron injections, Rick goes to the pharmacy to collect the fertility drugs and is handed a sturdy box of glass ampules. The amount of medicine seems so large that he telephones Cheryl from the parking lot to ask if there is some mistake. Cheryl calls the clinic and learns there's no mistake. Each ampule costs almost $50, and Cheryl requires seven ampules of medication a day. At the appointed time, Rick breaks open an ampule, always wary of the pieces of glass. Then he injects sterile water into the powder until it dissolves. He then draws the drug up into the syringe and injects the one-and-one-half-inch needle deep into the muscle of his wife's hip, offering comforting words and a hug when the injection is complete. Total cost of the ten-day dosage is $3,000. Rick put it on a charge card.

Once Cheryl starts the cycle, she is religious about the timing of the shots, sticking as close to the assigned hour as possible, a schedule that can turn an otherwise uneventful day upside down. They leave restaurants midmeal to get home on time. The skin on her hips and thighs soon feels lumpy and tender around the injection sites, and her tummy is black and blue. Cheryl says she feels like a human pincushion and cries through half the injections. Her teenage daughter cannot watch her mother feel so bad.

Rick is a stoic. He is firm and sure with each injection, talking to his wife throughout. Cheryl worries about his hitting a nerve accidentally during the deep intramuscular injections. She asks the nurse to draw big round circles on her rear so that Rick has the proper target. Other women bring their underwear into the clinic and have the nurse cut out a circle so they can clearly present the correct target. Rick begins giving Cheryl fertility drug injections in late November and doesn't hit a nerve once. But he worries about the amount of medication his wife is on.

Cheryl comes into the center seven days after the injections start for an ultrasound to monitor her follicles. I tell her she has forty-one follicles. They are small, 12 to 13 millimeters in size—too small to start the coast that day. The estrogen level in her blood is 4,220 pg/ml and climbing. But if I halt the fertility drugs now, the follicles would never be sufficiently mature, and the entire cycle would be lost. If she continues with the injections one more day, the follicles will be at 15 to 16 millimeters, perfect for initiating the coast. I explain this to her and tell her to return the following day.

The next day the follicles hit the correct size. By now, the level of estradiol has climbed to 7,300 pg/ml. So on December 6, we start the coast by stopping the injections of fertility drugs. But I tell the couple to continue with the injections of Lupron to hold off ovulation, and then we all wait and watch as Cheryl's estrogen level climbs, from 7,300 to 9,561 pg/ml. The next day it's 12,461, and then 13,329 pg/ml.

I seldom see estrogen levels that high. Without prolonged coasting, I'd have canceled Cheryl's cycle right at the first ultrasound; any doctor would do the same. But I'm confident we can get through these next few days without dangerous levels of hyperstimulation. Cheryl is concerned and keeps showing her swelling tummy to the nurse who performs her daily blood test. She starts reading fertility books, and what she sees on hyperstimulation terrifies her. It seems like everything that could possibly go wrong in a cycle is going wrong with her.

As I come out of my office a day later, I see Cheryl down the hall in the waiting room, crying. She has come in for her daily blood test while we're waiting for the estradiol to drop to a safe level. I hate to see Cheryl so upset and ask her to come back to speak to me.

"I'm huge," she said, crying and pointing to her abdomen where she had obviously begun retaining fluid. "And I'm scared that something awful is going to happen to me." I tell her that I know she is upset but that I can promise her the level of estrogen in her blood will drop and allow me to safely perform the retrieval and transfer. The levels finally come down after eight days, and I make good on the promise. The fluid retention will decrease over the next few weeks.

On December 14, Rick gives his wife the hCG, the final step in the stimulation, which allows us to schedule the egg retrieval. At the retrieval, Cheryl produces seventeen eggs. Three days later, she and Rick have eight good embryos. I am thrilled. All I can think is that we could have lost everything without the ability to do the prolonged coast.

Three days later, as I meet with them before the transfer, Cheryl is nervous. Rick, anticipating this, has brought mementos to help her relax. The transfer room reminds Rick of a massage therapy room—dim lights, the shush of a white noise machine, and a sense that something mysterious and special is taking place. He plays his wife's favorite music and throughout the procedure shows her flashcards made from photos of her older children when they were babies. Rick's pampering makes Cheryl giggle at one point, and she instantly becomes serious, worried that she's shaken the embryos loose. The nurse reassures her that this is not the case. The nurse reassures her that once the speculum is removed the cervix closes up, preventing the loss of her precious cargo.

I send the couple home. Cheryl continues to worry because she retains fluid in the two weeks after the transfer and her tummy is swollen. Rick worries, too, and wishes he had talked to me more about his concerns over the amount of the fertility drugs Cheryl has taken. He's especially upset because so many of the follicles failed to produce eggs. It's true that the process of coasting starves the granulosa cells around the eggs, causing some to die. At the same time, a woman needs to coast because she has already made at least two times the number of follicles than the average woman and so will have a healthy supply of eggs. But there is no question that some of the symptoms Cheryl is feeling are uncomfortable. I tell Cheryl to restrict her fluid intake to one liter of a sports drink a day and to measure her urine output to ensure there is not any potential for kidney failure. She is dying for a drink of water even with her distended tummy, and one night she can't help herself. She stands at the refrigerator and eats a lemon ice. It is the best thing she's ever tasted. It does no harm. A few weeks later her body has diffused the fluid she was retaining. Eight days after the transfer, Cheryl has a blood test done to detect pregnancy hormones in her blood; two days later, a second one is done to indicate whether the level of hormones has changed, which will determine if the pregnancy is progressing.

As I look back on the way Cheryl responded, I think that if I had to stimulate her again, I would probably back off a little on the fertility medication because she responded better than her elevated FSH level predicted she would. If you back off too much in a patient who has poly-cystic ovaries or is a known high responder, it is also easy to a have a much poorer response. The follicles will start to grow, but they seem to stall at the 10 mm size and the estrogen level stays low. Often their cycles then need to be canceled because of a poor response. High responders are so difficult to manage that it is one reason why many young women who respond vigorously are told that they have bad eggs when the prob-lem lies with the stimulation. Fortunately, we don't have to stimulate Cheryl again. The nurse gives this couple the news on the cellular phone while Rick and Cheryl are out running errands. They're pregnant!

It is a family affair, with Cheryl bringing her eleven-year-old son and her nineteen-year-old daughter into the office for her first sonogram. There are two gestational sacs obvious on the monitor, one with a fetal heartbeat. They all beam at the tiny pulse.

At seven weeks, Cheryl suffers one final scare. She is at home when cramps hit. As she walks toward the bathroom, blood begins flowing down her legs and all over the kitchen floor. She is hysterical. Rick comes running and carries her into the bathroom. They share with me the thought they both had at this point: All this to lose the baby.

When I get their panicked call I tell Cheryl not to assume anything, just to get to the office so that I can perform another ultrasound. On the monitor, one gestational sac is obvious. The heartbeat is fine; the baby is fine. I speculate that the bleeding was from the other sac detaching and passing in the most frightening way possible. But no matter what I say, it doesn't seem to quell the fear that will linger with Cheryl and Rick until she delivers the baby.

As with all my patients, at the end of Cheryl's twelfth week of preg-nancy, I say good-bye. At this point, I turn my patients' care over to their regular ob/gyn, who will monitor the rest of the pregnancy and deliver the baby. I wait for the baby announcement, and my staff teases me about my habit of writing "Congratulations!" in giant letters at the bot-tom of the patient's chart when that wonderful news arrives.

Postscript

"Congratulations!" I write on Cheryl and Rick's chart nearly twenty-eight weeks later. Baby Kristin was born on September 14, her father, Rick's birthday. She weighed just over nine pounds.

Rick had always said that if they never had more children, he was perfectly happy raising the two he and Cheryl already had. But once the family experienced the birth and presence of Kristin, he wondered how any of them had ever lived without her. Kristin was a dark-haired, round-cheeked blend of her parents. But she had eyes only for her big brother, whom she adored.

During the pregnancy, Cheryl endured other anxious moments—during the amniocentesis, which was fine; and during the labor, which was long. She worried when the baby developed a short, nasty infection after birth. Cheryl remembered the coasting portion of her cycle as among the most difficult periods of her adult life. Someday, Cheryl would like to write Kristin a letter telling her what they went through to have her and why. How the image of her kept them going. You have to wonder what kept Kristin going. Out of seventeen eggs, eight embryos, and two gestational sacs, she was the one who survived.

6 Pictures Don't Lie

Jamie's parents were among the most well-intentioned parents, acutely aware of proper manners, acceptable relationships, and the clear limits of polite society. So when one of their children crossed the line, they were firm, decisive, and immediately on the phone to the parish priest. This was known, in family circles, as the Father Moriarity response.

Their daughter, Jamie, had fortunately never attracted such intervention, living, as it were, an altogether exemplary life. She was pretty and very smart, working her way up at an investment firm where her level-headedness and thirty-foot putt were appreciated. She was a model daughter any parent would be proud of. Then, she fell in love with her boss.

For three years, William, a vice president of the investment firm, was an excellent supervisor to Jamie. The two worked together so compatibly that when other employees wanted his opinion on a subject, they simply began asking her. Sometimes she'd write memos, he'd sign them and then come back and say, "Did I write that?"

When his marriage ended, she was an equally efficient friend, advising him on apartments, and, occasionally, when he asked, she would step in loyally to accompany him to events that required a date.

Shortly after, the company began downsizing, and William was ordered to dismantle a division. He was so opposed to it that he added his own name to the list of people being laid off and left the firm. He quickly landed at a better firm, halfway across the country. The problem was: no Jamie. The void William's departure opened in both their lives was surprising to both of them and surprisingly deep. So, although they had never dated officially, they talked about this emptiness they felt and pretty much decided to get married. It took some time.

Jamie was twenty-eight and had never been married. William was almost forty and had been married—twice. He had two children who were closer in age to her than she was in age to him. When Jamie revealed the relationship to her parents, they saw his age and two divorces and responded immediately with the Father Moriarity response.

William decided to confront their disapproval head-on. He wrote Jamie's parents a long letter saying he understood their concern for their daughter but that he loved her and hoped they'd at least agree to meet him. Their response was not encouraging: "We pray to God every day that you will see your way clear to end this relationship."

When Jamie traveled home for the holiday, her parents were prepared: "We've made an appointment for you with Father Moriarity," they said. Jamie complied. She told the priest how a deep friendship between two professional colleagues had evolved into a deeper love. Father Moriarity listened carefully.

"I should be talking to your parents," he concluded when the conversation ended.

Friends advised Jamie and William to ignore her parents and elope. But that wasn't how either of them did business. The couple didn't want to start a marriage estranged from family. They returned to Jamie's home to visit Father Moriarity on their own to begin making wedding plans, and then called her parents back and asked them to meet for dinner.

Jamie introduced her fiancé to her parents at a tony restaurant Friday night and the conversation continued at the country club Saturday, where, in an empty dining room, the foursome squirmed under the lightness of what was said and the weight of what remained unsaid. Woody Allen couldn't have served up more tension.

Mercifully the weekend ended. As they were parting, Jamie's father snapped a photo of his daughter and the man she intended to marry.

Looking at the developed film several days later, Jamie's father had a dramatic change of heart.

"I've never seen her so happy," he told his wife.

That photograph, framed alongside a poem Jamie wrote, hangs in the hallway of William and Jamie's house. A copy of the photo is also framed above the kitchen sink. And in the bedroom, on the nightstand.

"Pictures don't lie," Jamie said.

The couple married at Jamie's parents' home with the help of Father Moriarity. Jamie had never really thought about being a wife and mother. But the more she enjoyed the one role, the more she envisioned the other.

Around her, thirty-something friends were so worried about their biological clocks, they seemed to be marrying just to have babies. They didn't marry the man, Jamie said, they married the sperm donor. She married the man, without question. She wanted William's children because of how she felt about him. But there was a problem.

William was a nineteen-year-old sophomore who married his college girlfriend when she became pregnant. After their second child was born, he had a vasectomy in 1975. He was twenty-four. The couple divorced a year later.

William attempted to have the sterilization reversed in 1987. One of the top urologists in the country performed a vasoepididymostomy in an effort to connect the vas deferens, the tube that carried sperm to the urethra, to the epididymis, the coiled network of tubes on top of each testicle where the sperm mature. The surgery failed. William's semen still had no sperm cells in it.

That knowledge put William and Jamie in a better position than many couples who are considering assisted reproduction. There was no mystery. They knew when they married that they would need help in order to have children. As a result, they weren't anguished by the infertility. They experienced almost none of the depression or self-recrimination that many of the couples I treat go through; Jamie and William knew there was a way to have a child; they just didn't know if that way included William.

When I meet Jamie and William in my office in November 1993, she is thirty and has never been pregnant. He is forty-two and has no sperm from the decades-old vasectomy and failed reversal. They want to know what assisted reproduction can offer as they consider their options for starting a family.

I told them that, at this point, they have two options: First, they could inseminate Jamie with donor sperm. Second, they could consider in vitro fertilization with intracytoplasmic sperm injection or ICSI, which involves the direct injection of a single sperm into an egg. For William to be the father, this would be effective only if his sperm was retrieved directly from his body with the additional procedure called testicular sperm extraction, or TESE. Attempts to use the micromanipulation technique on human eggs began in 1981, but its effectiveness in helping infertile couples was not fully realized until after a laboratory incident at the Free University in Brussels years later.

ICSI was about to become one of our most important tools. For years, men with low sperm counts or whose sperm had little forward motion had limited success even with in vitro fertilization. The problem was getting the sperm to penetrate the egg. The zona pellucida, the thick shell that protects the human egg, is a natural barrier that prevents more than one sperm from getting in. Normally, it takes millions of healthy sperm, moving in a forward motion, for one to penetrate the shell and have fertilization take place. Weak, deformed, or fewer sperm attempting to break through don't have a chance of breaching the barrier. Combining eggs and sperm with such conditions in a petri dish didn't seem to improve their chances.

For years, we tried using centrifuge and swim-up techniques to locate and concentrate the best sperm in order to overcome the zona pellucida barrier. It worked for some men with moderate problems but not for men with low sperm counts or defective sperm.

Then we looked at micromanipulation techniques to penetrate the zona pellucida. We tried softening the protective covering with enzymes and drilling through it with acids, slitting it open or injecting sperm through the zona pellucida but outside the cell membrane. It was during such a subzonal insemination procedure at the Free University in Brussels that a researcher noticed that one sperm had accidentally gone further and penetrated the cytoplasm. Hours later fertilization occurred. It renewed interest that one sperm could be effectively injected into the egg's center.

Researchers in Brussels quickly applied this technique to couples whose infertility was associated with low sperm count and motility, and four women became pregnant in 1992. One pregnancy ended in miscarriage. But the other three pregnancies produced two boys and a set of twins, a boy and a girl. What a revolution: We then knew fertilization of an egg no longer took an armada of sperm, it just took one little swimmer. As a result, couples who had male fertility issues responded in droves. Within four years, fifty thousand ICSI procedures would be performed worldwide.

Like most clinics in the United States in early 1994, we were doing ICSI, but not very well. We hadn't yet achieved a birth. Not until Frank Barnes arrived.

Barnes was a Missouri farm boy who went to the University of Wisconsin to study ways to improve his parents' farm back home near Independence. He became a Ph.D. embryologist who was successfully cloning cattle and performing gene therapy in cows in the late 1980s, years before a cloned sheep named Dolly made news.

Many of the leading minds in IVF and the techniques they developed for human treatment come directly from the animal sciences field. We call them the farm team. The competitiveness, research, and money in the livestock industry gave them something not available in human studies—massive practical experience.

Therefore, it was not so unusual that Barnes left the livestock industry in 1993 to work and train with in vitro pioneer Alan Trounson of Australia. Trounson was among the researchers who reported the world's first pregnancy from egg donation in 1983, and had most recently helped complete the study that produced one of the first pregnancies from an immature human egg. Barnes joined me in 1994 to supervise our laboratory.

When Barnes arrived, among the biggest challenges was perfecting the sheer mechanics of the process using equipment that combined German, Japanese, Swiss, and American technology. ICSI takes place entirely under a microscope. Using sophisticated micromanipulation tools, the fat round face of a mature egg is held immobile by suction. Then, an embryologist draws a single sperm—tail first—into a microscopic glass needle. The needle then pushes through the egg's shell into the cytoplasm, and the sperm is injected headfirst. Barnes also brought with him the confidence of his experience to perform the complex micromanipulation maneuvers and to train others how to do it. Most embryologists were scared to death they were going to kill the sperm and egg.

Barnes performed an ICSI case at our laboratory in San Francisco on November 15, 1994, and a pregnancy resulted. The child, a girl, was born in July 1995. Within a few short years, we'd be performing three hundred ICSI cases a year. By then a highly skilled embryologist in our lab would be able to inject an egg a minute. Despite all the practice, it would be the most physically and mentally intense sixty seconds ever seen in a laboratory. Embryologists are still scared to death of hurting the egg.

Is ICSI for everyone? No. If the sperm is normal and a woman has a lot of eggs, there is probably still an advantage to letting nature pick which sperm gets into the egg. But when I'm up against a sperm problem, I have no choice but to proceed with ICSI. And increasingly, we are using the technique in cases in which a couple has very few eggs available. We know ICSI will give us more fertilized eggs than we'd ever get letting the egg and sperm just fight it out.

ICSI has revolutionized fertility medicine, no question. We haven't cured male infertility, but we've certainly found a way to maneuver around it. Short-term studies have been reassuring, indicating that children born through ICSI have no more birth defects than the general population. Some researchers have reported an increased incidence of sex chromosome abnormalities, but the studies were so small, with only a handful of children, that the long-term implications and risks are unknown. It is reasonable to assume that if a man has a sperm problem because of a genetic defect he may pass that on to a male child through ICSI. I recommend that all men with severely impaired sperm function receive genetic counseling before proceeding with the technique. I feel with careful counseling of the parents and ongoing research we can continue to assess and understand these risks. We are finding more and more couples who benefit from ICSI.

The month after Frank Barnes conducts our first successful ICSI procedure, William and Jamie return to my office. It is December 1994. Two things happen to bring them in. First, Jamie starts a "life calendar" of goals, which makes them realize that to wait any longer is to have teenagers when William is in his middle sixties. They want to have two children in the next two years, or better yet, twins in the next year. Second, our center moved into their neighborhood at the base of Telegraph

Hill. The move to the Fisherman's Wharf area makes the undertaking seem very convenient. Jamie can walk to appointments.

In the months since William and Jamie first came to my office to learn their options, they've researched and shopped for clinics, insurance coverage, and information. They contacted sperm banks. They've decided to pursue in vitro fertilization with ICSI.

William has sperm, and a testicular biopsy confirms he has plenty of it. If we can get sperm cells directly from the testicle—whether they're motile or not—we can use ICSI to fertilize Jamie's eggs. Frank Barnes has the training to perform ICSI. The urologist who performed William's earlier biopsy knows how to perform testicular sperm extraction, which had been described in the medical journals earlier in 1994. We're also going to need donor sperm backup—insurance in case the procedure fails. Jamie and William have some hesitations about this, but we must have sperm available on the retrieval day if we are to fertilize the eggs. Of course, we hope it will be William's but we have to be prepared if the testicular extraction is not successful.

It's my job to bring all this together—and get the most and best eggs from Jamie to use in the ICSI procedure. I keep thinking of how many couples the combination of these procedures could help.

About 40 percent of the couples we treat have a sperm problem. It's either low sperm count, poor sperm movement, or abnormally shaped sperm. A small number of men have no sperm at all. Some are men born with a disorder that prevents them from producing sperm. Others are born missing the vas deferens, the tubes that connect the testes to the urethra. And others, like William, have had the vas deferens severed in a vasectomy to provide birth control.

For years, the only hope doctors could offer for a man with a vasectomy was microsurgery to reverse the operation. If it didn't work, some men underwent a second or even a third reversal.

In the mid-1980s, surgeons in St. Louis began to circumvent this obstacle by extracting sperm directly from the body. They could surgically remove sperm from the epididymis, the reservoir that contains the sperm before it reaches the vas deferens. Surgeons could also find sperm in the testes. But it was ICSI that made these techniques helpful for fertility treatment. No longer did you need millions of motile sperm, you just needed enough to find the right one.

There were other reasons why ICSI with in vitro fertilization could help William and Jamie. A curious thing happens in vasectomies. When the doctor severs the vas deferens from the testes, it prevents the sperm from reaching the ejaculate. A certain amount of sperm backs up in the body, triggering the body to produce antibodies to sperm. As a result, even when doctors successfully reverse the vasectomy, pregnancy may not result because of the actions of these antibodies. Antibodies make the sperm stick together, and clumped sperm can't penetrate the egg. More than 80 percent of men who had their vasectomy ten years or more before a fertility procedure will have high concentrations of these sperm antibodies. In fact, this is one reason why, in a few short years, TESE will be a good alternative for men whose vasectomies were performed five or ten years earlier. But, of course, this is 1994. We don't know that yet.

William tested 99 percent positive for sperm antibodies. Again, in vitro fertilization provides a way around this. Some doctors might prescribe steroids, such as prednisone, to temporarily suppress the antibodies' effects. Others will send patients to intrauterine insemination. I'm recommending IVF with ICSI because we know exactly how to ensure fertilization happens, despite any obstacles or the antibodies we'll face.

William and Jamie are ready and willing to go for it.

The key for all of this is going to be timing. On the morning of Jamie's egg retrieval, the urologist will perform a needle aspiration of William's testicle. Then, within two hours, we'll need to find the sperm in the tissue cells, carefully remove them, and send them to the ICSI table with Jamie's prepared eggs. I'm confident our plan will work. But to be safe, we need to have a donor sperm backup. We don't want to put Jamie through all this and then waste her eggs.

Intellectually, of course, and even emotionally, William and Jamie are open to using donor sperm. "It's not about the DNA," Jamie says. "It's about us being a family." But the reality of choosing a donor is something else. Files arrive in the mail from sperm banks, and Jamie spends hours reading pages that leave her feeling discouraged. "Why don't we know some great older man who could be the donor?" she writes in her journal. In her files—she has files on everything—she's collected stories of women infected with HIV through donor sperm before the discovery of HIV-AIDS. Jamie believes an older donor they knew would pose less of a risk. Her concern is understandable. The importance of using a disease-free sperm sample has been recognized from the very start of insemination. As early as the 1950s, when artificial insemination combined donor sperm and husband sperm, doctors demanded that donors be free of syphilis and other diseases, and have "unquestioned" mental health. It took the tragedy of AIDS to require the quarantine of all donated sperm. Since 1985, it has been recommended that all donor sperm be frozen six months first, so it can be tested for human immunodeficiency virus (HIV) and acquired immune deficiency syndrome (AIDS) before being used. Sperm is also tested for the Rh factor, hepatitis B and C, and other sexually transmitted diseases.

Jamie's anxiety reflects more unsettled feelings. The whole process of choosing a donor feels stranger and stranger to her. How do you pick someone based on the color of his eyes, height, complexion, weight, and occupation? Twice she liked donors only to turn the page and learn that both parents had died young of cancer or, in one case, a parent was living in a mental institution. She was grateful for the information, but it worried her.

"Who is this guy?" she asks William about candidates. "Why did he go in for this?" She wonders how William would be described by a sperm bank's staff: white; five feet, eleven inches; bedroom eyes? She ultimately picks the donor who looks as much like William as possible: similar height, weight, curly brown hair, and, yes, bedroom eyes.

In the time it has taken to reach this point, Jamie's sister and a single girlfriend have both become pregnant. Her mother keeps asking if she and William are ever going to have kids. Jamie tells her nothing about their plans.

As she and William prepare for a cycle in early 1995, Jamie tests positive for ureaplasma, a microorganism that can live in sperm or on a woman's cervix. It doesn't make people sick, but it can potentially interfere with egg implantation. As a result of these findings, I put them both on antibiotics and in ten days they should be good to go.

William gives his wife her first Lupron shot on Sunday, January 29. When the San Francisco 49ers beat San Diego in Superbowl XXIX the couple takes it as the best kind of sign.

William tries to keep the mood around the injections light. Each time he injects her, he asks, "What are our kids' names?" and she says,

"Molly, Megan, Michael, or David." Sometimes he gives her a little pinch in the rear so she won't know the needle is coming. The fact is, the process makes them think about becoming parents and renews their desire to have children. They never despair or feel sorry. It is their secret.

Jamie's response to the fertility drugs is phenomenal, and it becomes clear she has polycystic ovaries. Even two years earlier such a response would have forced us to cancel the cycle rather than risk sending Jamie into severe ovarian hyperstimulation. The sheer number of follicles Jamie has made could put her in real danger. But by using prolonged coasting, our technique to prevent severe hyperstimulation, we avoid serious complications. She may still feel some bloating and discomfort as her body begins to rest and recover after the retrieval.

On February 23, 1995, Jamie makes fifty-two eggs—I've seen only one patient produce more, a twenty-one-year-old woman who made fifty-six. I retrieve the eggs and send them to the laboratory. Now we need William's sperm. The urologist, operating in a procedure room at our clinic, takes four tissue core samples from William's testicle. It's an experience William describes as brief and painful, because of the amount of scar tissue from his earlier surgeries.

In a testicular sperm extraction, the slender cores of testicular tissue are finely minced, centrifuged, and treated in the laboratory. We get good news soon thereafter. There is motile sperm. William and Jamie are relieved to hear this and know they don't need to rely on the donor.

In the laboratory, embryologists spend the next few hours injecting each mature egg with a single sperm, an exhausting undertaking. First, it takes methodical searching to locate and separate the sperm cells, the smallest cells in the human body, from the testicular tissue. The sperm and egg are then prepared and taken to the ICSI table for the agonizingly precise work of injecting the sperm into the egg with a microscopic needle.

In vitro fertilization is nothing so much as the triumph of motor skills, a conquest of hand-to-eye coordination. From the retrieval of eggs to the injection of a single sperm into an egg, it is the victory of men and women over their own trembling hands.

After their procedures, Jamie and William both spend the next few hours resting. Three days later, on the morning of the transfer, we meet to discuss the couple's options. They have twelve embryos of widely varying quality. We transfer three of the best and five others that, by their very quality, have a much reduced chance of implanting.

Over the next few days, as we expected, fluid begins to accumulate in Jamie's abdomen due to hyperstimulation. She feels swollen and can't stand up without feeling sick. We restrict her fluid and watch her urine output; by late in the week, her symptoms begin to disappear. A woman who had not been coasted would have likely been in a life-threatening situation by now, as the symptoms of hyperstimulation reach a peak about seven days after the shot triggers the final step.

Jamie cannot tell whether she feels pregnant. The pregnancy test ten days later tells us she is not. The first blood test detected the faintest trace of pregnancy hormone, she likely had a nibble. But then, nothing. We can't believe it. Everything went as well as could be expected—we got good sperm and three excellent embryos. I'm asking myself what we can do differently. Is this just bad luck?

Jamie and William are grieving. If the problem was no sperm, and now with sperm Jamie still doesn't get pregnant, does that mean the problem is with her? The usually upbeat and philosophic woman is used to completing things, and her life now feels directionless; it is a series of stops and starts. They send a bill to their insurance company for $19,000 and learn insurance will cover just $10.

The couple is challenged by the disappointment and wants to try again—as soon as possible. I tell Jamie that her exhausted ovaries need a rest. I suggest she and William consider using the frozen embryos on the next cycle to spare herself the rigors of another stimulation. But Jamie knows it takes more frozen embryos to have the same success rate that a fresh cycle provides. They have only four embryos frozen from that attempt, and one or more may not survive the thaw. She wants to complete another fresh cycle.

"I'll be fine," she insists. "Now I know what to expect."

Looking at her response to the first cycle, I suggest decreasing the fertility drugs and I decide to add heparin and aspirin to her protocol.

Jamie and William proceed through their second cycle with determination. Their first attempt, with all its unfamiliar demands, felt like a science project. This time it feels much more like a conscious attempt to have a baby. Ultrasounds to monitor the progress of the stimulation indicate the process is going very well. And then, the bottom falls out.

Three days before the egg retrieval, a scheduling glitch with the urologist who was to perform William's testicular biopsy puts the doctor out of town during the scheduled retrieval. It's a fiasco. Unless we find a urologist who can perform this surgery, we will have to cancel the whole cycle, or rely on donor sperm. In reproduction, assisted or otherwise, timing is everything.

Then I remember Dr. Seck Chan, who had recently moved to San Francisco. He's an old friend who I first met in the early 1980s when he was in private practice in Vancouver and I was completing my fertility training at the University of British Columbia. Over the next ten years, we had a lot of patients in common. He would see the male partner in a couple while I evaluated the female partner. Chan had the best surgical hands in urology in Vancouver, but he also had impressive credentials in fertility medicine, having completed extra postgraduate work in Houston prior to going to Vancouver. Infertility had been an area ignored by many urologists when he first started, and the progress in treating people had been slow and frustrating. We had at one point actually talked about collaborating on testicular extraction cases but had never gotten together. Now, I need him, and my patient needs him desperately.

I telephone my old friend, and we meet for lunch. When I explain the predicament, Chan immediately offers to help. He meets William and Jamie the morning of the procedure. First, Chan prepped the scrotum with alcohol. Then, he deadened the area with a local anesthetic. Next, he used a spring-loaded needle biopsy gun to go in about 17 millimeters, about half an inch or so, into each of the four quadrants of William's testicle. Pressure was then applied to the area and ice for twenty minutes. Chan tells William to expect some discomfort for up to two days. The whole procedure takes less than thirty minutes.

The thin cores of testicular tissue that Chan extracted are sent to the laboratory where embryologists mince and centrifuge the sample to locate the sperm cells. The sperm are present and moving. "Swimmers," Jamie exalts. Meanwhile, she produces thirty-eight eggs in the retrieval, an excellent response. When she wakes up from the anesthetic, William is in the chair next to her. She asks how the biopsy went and how the doctor was. "Good," he says with a sheepish smile. "Dr. Death Grip."

But the next morning, it is maddening to find that less than a third of the eggs fertilized. Why is the fertilization rate so low? At this time we don't realize, although we soon would, that sperm taken straight from a testicle is not activated, as it is when it comes directly from the epididymis or ejaculate.

Soon, research would help us realize that, in order to make testicular sperm competent to be able to fertilize the egg, the embryologist must activate it in the laboratory, as nature does in the human body. This is done by almost crushing the neck of sperm with a needle before you draw the sperm up into the micropipette to perform ICSI. As soon as you crush the neck, you release calcium and set in motion the chain of events that makes the sperm competent to fertilize the egg. We needed, in other words, to arm the warhead. It's an infinitesimally small motion, done through micromanipulation tools. Once we realize this, fertilization rates for testicular sperm will leap to the same fertilization rates we see in other sperm—about 75 percent. But in May 1995, when we are working with William and Jamie, the fertilization rates remain low. Nonetheless, we get eight good embryos. On the morning of the nineteenth, we transfer five embryos and freeze the remaining three. Now, all we can do is wait.

Jamie writes in her journal: "The suspense is killing me." She has prayed each day of this whole process. The day her pregnancy test results come back, she has gone with William while he golfs, and they telephone the center from the car phone.

"You are very pregnant," the nurse says. The amount of pregnancy hormone is high enough to suggest a multiple. It is Memorial Day—memorable for them and for all of us. This is our first pregnancy with testicular sperm extraction. We did it, with Seck Chan and Frank Barnes's help. Jamie and William are very excited.

An ultrasound scan a month later reveals three embryos have implanted. One gestational sac is quite small and doesn't appear to have a fetal pole, the mass of cells that constitute the early embryo that becomes the baby. Jamie prays it reabsorbs. At ten weeks, when we look at the ultrasound monitor, the smallest embryo sac is gone and the other two are growing nicely.

"There's the little munchkin, and there's the other one," I say. Twins. Exactly what they wanted. She and William are very happy; it feels as if what is happening is exactly right. Jamie calls me a few hours later with just one question! Can she still golf with her husband?

Yes, I reply, but I don't want her walking miles and miles, and I want her to be very careful with any rotational movement. What the pregnancy adds to her life is obvious even in her swing. She golfs the best game of her life at five months.

Postscript

At thirty-nine weeks, Jamie delivered twin girls, Molly at six pounds, six ounces, and Megan at six pounds, three ounces. The twins' birth was the first TESE pregnancy our clinic recorded. Since then, Chan and our staff have performed more than five hundred TESE procedures. ICSI continues to offer consistent rates of success for couples with male factor infertility or few eggs. Jamie and William's pregnancy made headlines in California and the evening news. Thousands learned of their achievement. But Jamie's parents don't know. They never will.

"It was the greatest decision I ever made," Jamie said. "They don't know now, and I'll never tell them."

She didn't tell them because she thought they would have worried too much during the pregnancy and would always be expecting the children to begin walking funny once they were born. William's family, on the other hand, knows everything. His divorce as a young man made him a weekend father for his older children, and the birth of the twins forced them all to confront the pain they experienced from that time. He took a different job to spend more time at home with Jamie and the kids, and is contemplating early retirement. He is the father now that he wished he could have been for his older children.

The twins are magic. They have blond ringlets and angel faces. And you see their little mugs all over Jamie and William's house. When they were pregnant, a nurse at our center told them that they should photograph the children in the same spot in their house every month, as a chronicle of their potential, growth, and addition to the family. The pictures are displayed alongside the photos that convinced Jamie's parents that she belonged with William. Pictures don't lie.

7 The Bleeding Edge

There was talk that year in Jersey.

"Hey, have you seen Joe and Judith around? Where those guys been? Everything okay with those guys? Geez. They're always gone anymore. Going here, going there, off to San Francisco. What a life. They got it made, eh? Old Joey, he did okay for himself, a Jersey City kid. He's done all right. Tough life those two have, huh? It's January, and they're on vacation."

Joe hung on to other people like other people hung on to real estate. He had the same best friend for thirty-three years. The same attorney for twenty-three years and the same accountant. He fell for one girl, and they're still married. If people mattered at all in his life, they stayed.

Jersey City, where he grew up, was nobody's idea of beachfront. It was gritty and smoky and poor. He grew up in a family of five in a two-room apartment. His father cleaned city parks, his mother cleaned houses, and he was the first one in his family to see the way out.

One afternoon his parochial school principal called looking for him, and his father, who answered the telephone, lied. "Joe is sick in bed." When Joe came home, his father was waiting. His father spoke Ukrainian at home.

Where you been?

He'd been to the New York Stock Exchange. When he was still in grammar school, Joe would skip classes to catch the ferry across to Wall Street. In those days, before security glass and cellular telephones, he'd talk his way onto the Stock Exchange floor where the shouting and signaling opened his eyes to the mystery and power of money, a magic kingdom.

To Joe, it was all about relationships. If a trader gave his word, he stuck to it or he'd be out of a reputation and likely out of a job. If a trader changed his mind on a deal, he swallowed hard. Traders did what they said they would. This a Jersey City kid could understand.

He studied engineering in college because he was good with numbers, and he played on the university's basketball team where his game was about numbers, too. If he kept putting the ball up, he figured it eventually would go in.

He had a friend—still his best friend—who knew a dark-haired, dark-eyed woman named Judith who was very pretty and very smart. The friend forgot to mention that she was ice-cold. Joe called her for more than two months, and while she would talk to him, she wouldn't agree to meet him.

One night he learned she was in East Orange shooting pool with a girlfriend. Joe showed up at the next table dropping combination shots and come-ons. Her girlfriend was more interested than Judith, who kept thinking, Who is this guy?

When Judith got home, the telephone rang. It was Joe asking to come over. She finally said yes, and when she opened the door, she recognized the pool player from the next table as the Joe she'd been talking to on the telephone for months. Joe couldn't possibly have known that the woman before him had already decided she would marry him. She made up her mind during one of their long phone conversations before they ever met in person. It was when she told him one weekend that she would be driving to Philly in a snowstorm. He said he'd come to get her if she ran into trouble. And she knew he would. She thought: This is a man who solved problems, who, when trouble hit, would stick around. They married when they were twenty-five.

They worked hard: He tackled industrial engineering and then the construction business; she finished her degrees and built a practice in psychotherapy. Clients who moved away called her from all over the country. She nurtured a lot of troubled souls. There was never a decision not to have children. The decision was always about when. As a couple, they always seemed to take longer than their friends to get somewhere, to finish college, to marry, to start a family. It took them sixteen years to buy their first house.

Then, approaching forty, Joe got sick. He was hospitalized several times with intestinal blockages caused by an operation he'd had as an infant. After he recovered, Judith wanted nothing as much as to build a fortress, to make him impervious to sickness and death. She wanted to have his children. That she was almost forty never entered her mind. Nobody was using the phrase "biological clock" back then, and Joe and Judith certainly didn't know their clock was ticking away.

They decided, finally, that it was time to try to have a baby. When nothing happened, they went to one doctor, then another, from artificial insemination to fertility drugs with intrauterine insemination. She got pregnant right away. She got pregnant at forty-two and at forty-three. And at forty-four.

Each pregnancy began with hope and excitement. Each one ended within nine weeks. There would be no outward sign that the pregnancy had ended. She'd go in for an ultrasound full of hope, and the doctor would point out a gestational sac and then in the silence it would become obvious that there was no fetal heartbeat or fetal pole inside. The fetal pole, the mass of cells that constitutes the early embryo that then becomes the baby, is about the size of a grain of rice at five weeks; at six weeks, the heartbeat can be detected in its midst by ultrasound. The gestational sac Judith saw would be empty or, worse, would contain what the doctor called "debris." The technical term used was "blighted ovum," and Judith became what is known as a "habitual aborter."

How much easier it would have been just to discover blood at home in the bathroom. Judith never had the luxury of private grief.

The fertility doctors the couple visited began increasingly to point to her age, hinting, if not saying flat out, that she had passed the open window. Judith and Joe knew they were viewed as a drag on a fertility program's success rates. They ignored message after not-so-subtle message to give up. Many programs would not accept women over forty-two and by then she was four years past that. The couple kept looking for help. When a doctor suspected Judith's immune system was rejecting the pregnancies, she and Joe drove back down to Philly where she underwent paternal leukocyte immunization or lymphocyte immune therapy (LIT). To the body, a pregnancy can look like an invader. The baby a woman carries is an immunologic foreigner, the surface of the early embryo expresses almost exclusively the sperm provider's genetics. Normally, the mother's body recognizes the implanting embryo and produces friendly blocking antibodies to protect it. But sometimes this mechanism breaks down and the embryo may no longer be protected from rejection.

A decade earlier, Dr. Alan Beer of Chicago was among the first to theorize that some women's bodies fail to develop the blocking antibodies because their immune systems are so similar genetically to the father's. Their bodies do not recognize the embryo as sufficiently different. As the embryo grows, it is not protected by the special blocking antibodies and is attacked by her immune system and dies. Beer and others began treating women with recurrent miscarriage for this deficiency by immunizing them with white blood cells from their partners. Joe's white cells were purified and injected into Judith's arm until her system recognized his antigens and developed the necessary antibodies. Judith underwent the procedure, but nothing different happened.

Judith still got her period, and the hormone levels in her blood were normal, but the age of her eggs was finally catching up with her. Her ob/gyn said that while she may be producing eggs—and may even get healthy-appearing embryos—the chances of one of those embryos growing into a healthy, normal baby were slipping to a fraction of a percent. Her doctor told her she needed to consider donor eggs.

For many women, this is the sound of a door closing, the end of a dream of being a genetic mother, a mom. However, Judith felt only enormous relief. Even if her body couldn't produce eggs, she could still have the experience of being pregnant and raising a child. She could still carry what she wanted most, a part of Joe.

By 1993, egg donation was becoming more available nationwide. Some of the most successful programs were in California, where in the laid-back, liberal, and entrepreneurial air, anonymous donors were compensated for their time and risk. The attitude extended to fertility doctors, who didn't blink at a woman over forty. Judith's East Coast doctor referred her to one West Coast facility where this procedure was performed regularly with mature women. This is how they came to San Francisco.

Judith and Joe got ready for an in vitro fertilization cycle, taking everything from blood tests to psychological exams long distance. They contacted three agencies specializing in egg donors and, after quantifying and qualifying the profiles of twenty young women, made their selection. Joe, who quantifies most things, noted that more than half of the candidates were of Irish descent.

The first donor they chose dropped out after learning the extent of the injections. The second donor was an attorney who completed the preparation to donate her eggs. In November, Judith and Joe flew to San Francisco for a cycle with one of my former partners. When the lining of Judith's uterus was the proper thickness, thanks to hormone injections, I scheduled the donor's egg retrieval and retrieved thirteen eggs. They were fertilized with Joe's sperm that morning and three days later, a catheter containing six embryos was threaded through Judith's cervix and the embryos injected.

None implanted. Her San Francisco doctor at that time attributed the failed cycle to "bad luck." Another cycle, scheduled for January, was performed with frozen embryos from the first cycle. The couple flew home to New Jersey, where they learned that another pregnancy test was negative. More bad luck.

Doctors' notes from the time say Judith telephoned sounding concerned and depressed. But no one at home guessed that the couple was doing in vitro fertilization cycles on the side, compartmentalizing their trips and treatment, separating it completely from the rest of their lives. The shots and schedules and payments were in a parallel universe. It was too hard for them to talk about, the disappointment too hard to share. Shortly after their last cycle, for instance, Judith discovered their egg donor had gone on to help another couple. That couple was now expecting.

It's me, it's me, Judith kept hearing a voice say inside. There's something wrong with me.

Judith and Joe arrive in San Francisco on July 4, 1994, before the fireworks but after the parade. I'm the medical director of our San Francisco office and the surgeon who performs laparoscopies. I've been consulted to help determine whether Judith's implantation problems may be related to two fibroids in her uterus. Joe and Judith and their new donor are on the verge of an egg retrieval, and we need to decide today whether to proceed with a transfer of fresh embryos or to perform fibroid surgery and freeze the embryos for later use. On the basis of the discovery of a third and far larger fibroid, I vote for surgery.

Fibroids look a little like the inside of a golf ball, layers of fibrous tissue wrapped around other layers. They grow in or around the uterine cavity and can cause bleeding, become inflamed, and press on the bladder and rectum. The most common are subserous fibroids, which grow just beneath the outer layer of the uterus. Intramural fibroids grow in the muscular walls, and submucous fibroids, the rarest kind, grow under the uterine lining. It turns out Judith has all three kinds. Many women with fibroids have no symptoms. But for the woman trying to conceive, fibroids can interfere with the embryo's ability to implant, negatively affecting the lining of the uterus or even blocking the fallopian tubes. Because fibroids grow in response to estrogen, they can also grow during pregnancy and compete with the baby's blood supply, causing miscarriage and premature birth. Most fibroids shrink at menopause. We are going to shrink the fibroids as much as possible before surgery by putting Judith in a near-menopausal state with injections of Lupron, which suppresses her own hormone production.

On August 10, I schedule a laparoscopy to remove what I believe are two or three fibroids. Looking through the long, thin telescope inserted through Judith's navel, I'm surprised to discover seven. The masses of tissue range from a half-inch in size to an inch and a half in size. The largest, No. 5, is protruding about 30 percent into the uterine cavity from the back wall. This is a problem. To reach it, I'm going to have to go into the cavity. The incision will weaken the uterine wall sufficiently that, if Judith becomes pregnant, she'll need a cesarean section. But the fibroid's sheer size and location leave me no choice other than to remove it. If Judith and Joe want the best chance to have a baby, that fibroid needs to come out. The laparoscopic surgery goes well, and the day after I perform it, Judith leaves the hospital.

Late that fall Judith and Joe arrive in San Francisco once again to transfer the embryos we fertilized and froze the summer before. Whenever we talk, Joe wants numbers, he wants a way to quantify their chances. At this point, we think their chances look good. Judith's uterus looks beautiful and normal, it is perfectly healed. She's been taking shots of estrogen and progesterone, and, on the ultrasound monitor, the rich nurturing lining of the uterus looks just as it should at this stage.

Six of the embryos we froze from the summer cycle are thawed and are growing nicely. We transfer all six in the procedure room in our new office.

Ten days later, the pregnancy test shows the hormone in Judith's blood rises. Then drops, then disappears.

In assisted reproduction, a woman can be a little bit pregnant. An embryo can implant, triggering her hormones and registering what we call a "chemical pregnancy," but the embryo never flourishes. It probably happens all the time in nature, and most people never know it. But in assisted reproduction we are watching and waiting for the faintest nibble. Losing a pregnancy, even one just days old, is a loss, a frustration, and a disappointment. I telephone Judith and Joe to discuss it, in what will become the first of the "Tiburon talks."

Tiburon is an exclusive community north of San Francisco in Marin County. I don't live there; I live several exits north. But I often speak to Judith and Joe as I'm passing it on my drive home from work. It's 10 P.M. Eastern Standard Time, and they're usually both home. My long commute gives us a chance to talk.

What happened? they ask. The donated eggs were twenty-five years old, and the embryos were well divided and of very good quality, so we're probably not dealing with an egg problem, I say. Judith has become pregnant and lost her pregnancy four different times. I think that, on the basis of these clues, it has to be an immune problem, which means antibodies and/or cells are somehow working against implantation.

Judith is already using heparin and aspirin. Her NK assay shows increased activity, suggesting that the cellular side of her immune system is also being directed against the implanting embryos. I think that we need to consider using the immunoglobulin, IVIG. The use of this purified human blood product is a controversial therapy for patients with repeated pregnancy loss or repeated failed IVF attempts.

I believe that there is a subset of patients with recurrent miscarriage and IVF failures who require immunotherapy in order to establish and nurture a pregnancy to successful delivery. There are no large prospective randomized studies to support this therapy, but the fact of the matter is, it is inordinately difficult to recruit patients who have been brutalized by repeated loss and failure into the very studies that are needed to validate this therapy in the eyes of the general scientific community. However, a strong body of evidence exists from case studies and from the successful therapy of noninfertility patients who have had recurrent miscarriages and then, with the correct immunotherapy such as IVIG and LIT, went on to have a delivery rate of 85 percent with their next spontaneous pregnancy. I believe the results of this immunotherapy can be extrapolated to infertility patients with repeated pregnancy loss and repeated IVF failure.

How IVIG works is not totally clear. In the broadest sense, IVIG behaves like an anti-inflammatory agent regulating the NK cell activity and possibly supplying friendly blocking antibodies. In the years to come, data from Dr. Alan Beer confirms that leukocyte immunization therapy alone may decrease the natural killer activity by 50 percent, thereby making IVIG unnecessary for some patients, and reducing the total dose of IVIG required for other, more difficult cases.

Joe's onboard with our plan to address Judith's immune system. He's philosophical about their chances and upbeat. He is convinced we will find our way to a baby. Judith is less convinced. Her voice sounds distant, and I don't think it's because of the car phone.

In May, her egg donor begins taking fertility drugs on the West Coast while Judith begins preparing her uterus on the East Coast with the drug protocol we've discussed and launched. We all move toward a transfer at the end of June.

I see this as the Olympics of reproduction. Hours and hours of tests and preparation and care all leading up to a few precious moments: The Event. In the hectic days before the transfer, Joe gives his wife shots of estrogen, in the form of estradiol valerate, twice a week, and progesterone daily. She gets a shot of heparin in the stomach every twelve hours and chews and swallows a baby aspirin tablet each morning. We're pumping up her hormone shots and giving her vaginal suppositories to plump up her uterine lining a bit. And right before the transfer we'll give Judith IVIG. The regimen is so intense that most people design charts and create files or envelopes to keep track of the pills and shots and timing. The paper trail buries desks and dining room tables.

The week before their flight west on June 26 for the transfer, Judith is brought up sharply by stomach pain. Sharp, breath-crushing pain. She goes to the doctor, who schedules laparoscopic surgery immediately to remove a "hot gallbladder." Joe calls our office a bit panicked: How will gallbladder surgery at the beginning of the week affect a transfer the following weekend? As long as everything goes well, I don't know why she can't make it out here by the weekend to proceed, I tell him. We stop her clotting medication immediately and wish her well.

But nothing goes well. Judith has her gallbladder removed Monday. By Wednesday, her abdomen is so tender she cannot straighten. As she's being wheeled out of the hospital, she complains of shooting pain. For the first time in their marriage, Joe has disappeared when she really needs him. She is at her parents' house that afternoon, barely able to breathe for the pain, when he returns.

"We have to go back to the hospital," she gasps.

Joe calls me shortly after he takes her in. I know Judith has a high pain threshold, judging from the fibroid removal I performed. If they readmit her for abdominal pain, my guess is that she has a bile leak.

In fact, she does. When removing her gallbladder, the surgeon accidentally nicked Judith's common bile duct, and bile is spilling into her abdominal cavity with potentially lethal consequences. That night, major abdominal surgery is performed, and a drainage tube is inserted. Three thousand miles away, her egg donor has already taken the shot that triggers ovulation. The egg retrieval, at this point, must go on.

Judith and Joe are in a real spot. Judith has had two major surgeries in four days, and will be in the hospital for at least four more days. The eggs will be ready the day after tomorrow. We can salvage the cycle only if the eggs are fertilized within eight hours of the retrieval. But we need Joe's sperm to do it. If Joe cannot get to San Francisco in a day to provide semen, the eggs I retrieve will be lost.

Human eggs should be inseminated two to six hours after they are retrieved from the donor's ovaries. The timing is so critical that we insist each intended father provide sperm twice. We have him produce sperm two days before the retrieval so we can freeze it as a backup in case anything prevents him from producing on the critical day. Obstacles do come up: People get stuck in traffic, they get sick, they get inhibited and can't produce. Without sperm, we have no fertilization; without fertilization, we have no embryos; without embryos, we have no transfer. And at this point, in 1995, we have no way to cryopreserve eggs.

Joe has to get to San Francisco before the retrieval, or months of preparation and money will be lost. He spends the night nodding off on the hospital windowsill next to Judith's bed, where she lies seriously ill. He heads to the airport before sunrise to catch the first plane out. He flies standby and has to talk his way onto the airplane.

"I have to be on this flight, it's a medical emergency, I have to deliver something. I have to deliver it personally," he keeps saying at the ticket counter. At the last minute, he's allowed to board the plane. Joe blows into our clinic almost ten hours later, just in time to get into the room we call the Oval Office to produce his sperm sample for the insemination.

It is a year to the day since we first met. Joe is a dynamite sperm pro-ducer; his sperm has been consistently numerous, motile, and well formed. But he has taken a bit of a beating in the last seventy-two hours. His sperm count drops to about half what it was in previous samples, and the volume is down by three-quarters. This man is stressed. Still, I see that his production is so high that the sample is still in the nor-mal range. In the laboratory, the embryologist mixes his sperm with the donor's eggs and the following morning reports that Judith and Joe have seventeen embryos. After two days of growth in the laboratory, there are eleven excellent embryos and six more good ones. We freeze them all for a future transfer. Joe, spent, is already on his way back home.

Ten days later, Judith is home recovering when she opens a letter from their insurance company. While she was undergoing emergency surgery, their summerhouse caught fire and burned to the ground. Apparently, the day she had her gallbladder removed, the cleaning ser-vice, picking up after renters, stuffed the clothes dryer with wet towels, turned the dryer on, and left. The overworked dryer caused a fire. By the time the fire department arrived, the interior was gutted. Joe was myste-riously absent the day she left the hospital, because he had been called out to the scene to see the damage.

"When were you going to tell me?" she demands.

"When you were feeling better," he says.

What a summer. Within ten days, she had had two major surgeries, lost a home, and almost lost their chance at a baby. A more superstitious woman would have taken this as a sign. Judith forges ahead.

But it takes a long time for them to recover. Judith's body does not immediately bounce back from the operations, and she and her hus-band are distracted with rebuilding their summer home and with a move into a new house they'd been planning for some time. Not until February can Judith travel to see me on the West Coast to undergo the transfer of the embryos.

Judith has not had a period since the gallbladder surgery. She is defi-nitely menopausal, but that will not affect the coming cycle. Because we supply the estrogen and progesterone needed to maintain the pregnancy, she doesn't even need her ovaries. She needs just what she has—a healthy uterus.

The cycle is scheduled for the first week of February. The preparation for The Event begins again. But the night before the couple leaves for San Francisco, a massive winter storm dumps several feet of snow on the Northeast. Judith calls the center worried sick. The embryos we are planning to transfer can survive only a short time in the laboratory. If their flight gets delayed en route, all their embryos will be lost. I direct the laboratory staff to hold off thawing the embryos until I get the sign that they're going to arrive. On their way to the airport, Joe and Judith get a flat tire alongside an icy road in New Jersey. Joe changes the tire in a snowbank, where he loses the sole of his shoe. Hours later, they limp into San Francisco.

Judith is six months older. She has had two major surgeries and two major moves since the first transfer. The stress on her and her husband has been immense. The quality of frozen embryos is not as good as that of fresh. We decide that her best chances lie with transferring eight embryos.

This has been the craziest possible roller coaster, but it is all about to be worth it.

"Congratulations," says the nurse who reaches the couple at home ten days later. "The tests tell us you are pregnant at this time." We ship a package of medication and additional suppositories immediately to continue to boost her hormones. She has undergone an infusion of immunoglobulin and is injecting heparin into her stomach every twelve hours. A nurse encloses a note: "You're on your way!" Judith feels pregnant.

At six weeks, Judith and Joe, both anxious and hopeful, go into their local doctor for the ultrasound examination. When a strange and sudden silence develops in the room, Judith knows, with a withering certainty, that the pregnancy is done. The little embryo that had started to grow has just disappeared. It takes everything Judith has to stand up again.

I'm on the freeway nearly at the Tiburon exit in bad traffic when I get them on the telephone. For a moment, I cannot think of a single thing to say. Judith is struggling not to scream, struggling to be rational, but what she really wants to do is wail, "Tell me why this happened." And, of course, I can't. I don't know. The three of us don't have an answer. Judith and Joe are both trying to cope with catastrophic news when they have already had two catastrophes during the previous two cycles.

"There is just something weird with me," Judith says in a flat voice. She is expecting me to agree and to tell her that we've done everything we can.

But I won't. Obviously something has just wiped out this pregnancy. We've been using immunotherapy, which seems aggressive because most clinics do not use it. But now we have to become *truly* aggressive. Typically, when we add immunoglobulin to a patient's protocol, we pick an amount, stick with it, and either get a baby or not. I think we can do more. I can customize Judith's treatment. We can double the dose of IVIG, keep her on her prednisone, and monitor her immunotherapy weekly, making adjustments whenever necessary. I tell them this.

Joe says it's an old marketing technique: When a new product replaces an old product, you want the new one coming in as the other is petering out. You don't wait until the shelves are empty. It's an excellent analogy for how we're going to use the IVIG. We don't want the levels dropping off before the next infusion; we want a steady level, and we agree that means an infusion every three weeks. After everything Joe and Judith have been through, I feel we are going to find a way.

Judith and Joe are almost fifty. Many people, if they knew of this, would be screaming for all of us involved to stop. They would say we are fighting Father Time, violating Mother Nature's rules. David Thomasma, Ph.D., professor and director of the Medical Humanities Program at Loyola University, Chicago Medical Center, would tell those people that their argument is weak. As humans we try to improve on nature all the time, from the strength of steel bridges to tomatoes that can survive shipment from southern states to Alaska. We have air-conditioning, for goodness sake. Many of the most respected ethicists in the world are concerned about helping post-menopausal women become mothers. A more understandable concern is whether the women who want to bear children at this age are sufficiently healthy to carry and nurture a baby. Judith is. One of the first principles Thomasma and other members of our ethics advisory board helped our staff establish is to produce the best possible baby in the best possible environment.

Age doesn't destroy a happy home. Hundreds of thousands of people are the successful products of their grandparents' rearing. In my experience with thousands of families over the last fifteen years, older parents bring wonderful mature life skills to their parenting. They bring far more financial security, emotional stability, and attention than a distracted twenty-two-year-old.

Judith might well be the mother of a ten-year-old now if we had only been able to help her have a child when she began trying a decade ago. Her whole treatment has taken place on a vast learning curve that is pushing the science forward. She has been on the edge of that curve, what Joe calls the bleeding edge, this whole time.

Judith never wanted to parent in order to pass a part of herself along. She wants a baby so the world will have more of Joe, and because she knew that he would be an uncommonly good father. He takes care of people. He stays in place. I smile at Judith when she makes this disclosure because I know Joe wants a baby to see the mother in her. Maybe only people with their peculiar chemistry would keep pressing on in the face of such adversity. Maybe only kids who learned to play the game on a cracked and weedy asphalt court.

"You throw up a shot and miss, but if you keep throwing up another and another, eventually you'll make it," Joe says. "It's true with basketball and true with life."

Having used all their frozen embryos, the couple decides to undergo a fresh cycle with a new egg donor. Years before, they had quite a system for scoring and quantifying candidates: giving a candidate a "3" for good health, a "4" for higher education, adding the qualities up to determine the best choice of egg donor. Not this time. This time, they go with their gut. They read the profiles of donor candidates independently, each name their first choice, and are not surprised to find they've picked the same woman. There is something about her face and what she wrote about herself that just seems honest, straightforward, and lovely, Judith says. It's not that she's beautiful; it's that she has exactly the right look.

I arrange for their transfer in January.

A week before the scheduled procedure, I get a message that another panicked call has come from Judith and Joe. Judith was supposed to take 2 milligrams of estrogen, and then, four days later, take 4 milligrams. But Joe, the numbers man, has mistakenly given her 20 milligrams, and two days later, 40 milligrams. In other words, he gave her ten times the prescribed dose. Twice. He is mortified. Mortified that the stress has obviously gotten to him. Mortified that he could have accidentally done something to hurt her. I call them back immediately.

"First of all, you've taken way too much estrogen," I tell Judith. Fortunately it's not seriously detrimental. I tell her to skip the next dose and we'll watch her blood tests closely to determine how much she should take from then on. Her breasts will be tender, and she may feel nauseous, but there should be no serious long-term effects. High levels of estrogen can cause blood-clotting problems as well, but since Judith is taking the blood thinners heparin and aspirin in preparation for the transfer, I'm not as concerned that this will happen.

This type of mistake happens more frequently than one would expect. The protocols we use are complex. Patients are under extremely intense schedules, juggling two and three different injections a day. One reason patients need good emotional support at home, and twenty-four-hour telephone access to the center, is because everyone occasionally goofs up. I can think of at least six patients who have done exactly the same thing with the estrogen shots, and, interestingly enough, five of them became pregnant.

A week later, Judith and Joe arrive, on time, in San Francisco. Joe comes into the center to produce his backup sperm sample. His numbers and volume have returned to their normal level. Three days later, we meet in my office to discuss the embryo report from the laboratory. It's excellent. After Joe's sperm are mixed with the donor's eggs, they have twenty embryos. The embryologist reports that more than half of the embryos are flawless. These are stellar embryos and certainly have the best chance of implanting.

We decide to transfer six. This is aggressive, but Judith has lost five pregnancies so far. In two months, she will be fifty-one years old. We're also going to have the laboratory do assisted hatching on all six. In this procedure, the egg's translucent shell is thinned to help the embryo break out or hatch. We are marshaling every force we can think of to help an embryo implant and grow. Joe recognizes the strategy from basketball; it's what he'd call a full-court press.

On the morning of the transfer, Joe and Judith are in the procedure room talking quietly. The embryo transfer consists of a series of highly formal and methodical steps. In each procedure, the embryos are carried from the laboratory in a sealed Edwards-Wallace catheter. Judith's cervix is rinsed with the same culture fluid the embryos have been growing in, thus promoting some continuity in their environment. The catheter containing the embryos is then threaded through the cervix to a prescribed depth, about 5 millimeters from the top of her uterus.

"Transfer the embryos," I say, and the embryologist presses on the syringe, so that the fluid and the embryos are discharged. A second embryologist clicks a stopwatch. We wait thirty seconds, and then I slowly withdraw the catheter, turning it through two complete revolutions. I want the catheter to spiral so that if the embryos try to follow the catheter out, they get caught in the vortex. I hand the catheter back to the two embryologists. They return to the laboratory to examine any contents still within under the microscope, thus ensuring that all the embryos have been discharged.

We wait in silence. These few minutes are a solemn time, a very introspective time, and for most people a very sacred time. We are returning a couple's genetic material to them in the hopes that one or two embryos implant.

We perform eighty transfers like this a month and in one or two cases the embryologist will return to say that one embryo has refluxed and remains in the catheter. This morning is one of those times. Judith, I say, we have two choices. We can take out the speculum and you can rest, or we can just wait as we are and the lab will bring the embryo back in four or five minutes. They have to put the little guy in fluid again and draw it into a fresh catheter. Judith says she can wait. Joe asks if there is anything harmful about putting an embryo in after the fact. I tell him our data suggest that that does not seem to have a measurable detrimental effect.

When the two embryologists return, I thread the catheter back to the prescribed depth of 67 millimeters and repeat the process exactly as before. This time when the embryologist returns, she says, "All clear."

Maybe tenacity is genetic. Maybe the sheer stick-to-itiveness reminds Judith of Joe's tendency to hang on. But there is a part of Judith that recognizes the last embryo that clung to the catheter. She knows in her marrow that that last embryo is her son, Jon.

Postscript

Judith is in the examination room again with her husband and her doctor and the unblinking eye of the ultrasound monitor. I wanted her to wait a few more weeks. I don't want her to have an ultrasound scan so early that she might see a sac but no heartbeat. But she started bleeding two nights ago, and she is too sad, too scared to wait any longer. So here she is in the ultrasound examining room again, dying to know, just dying.

There are two gestational sacs, the doctor says. One is empty. One is not. The second one has the faintest heartbeat, a flutter. By nine weeks and four days, it's a strong pulse.

Judith walks around for the next several months consciously trying to squeeze everything in her pelvic area together; she's willing the baby to hang on. The pregnancy progresses, a small miracle, without morning sickness, nausea, swelling, or gestational diabetes. She takes long walks and goes to work and feels wonderful. When she and Joe slowly start telling people they are expecting, nobody can believe they had this secret.

The best friend who introduced them choked when hearing the news over dinner. Friends had her pegged as an all-career woman. They took Joe as all capitalist. They were dumbstruck.

The baby, a son, was born on an autumn afternoon, seven pounds, six ounces, making Joe's mother a grandmother for the first time at eighty-six. Judith and Joe are old enough themselves to be grandparents. The debate over treating post-menopausal women includes the argument that it creates orphans, children who in fifteen years may be all alone. Joe and Judith are painfully aware they may die before their son reaches thirty, or even twenty. They are doing their best to ensure through friends and relatives that a loving extended family will be there for him.

If I had one wish, it would be to have an old head on a young body. The tragedy of life is that as the head and wisdom improve, the body crumbles. Everything this couple does illustrates their caring and concern for their son now and in the years ahead. Joe has changed a lifetime of work habits to spend more time at home with Jon, feeding and caring for him. But the last bottle of the day belongs to Judith. Each night she

takes the baby in her arms, rocking while he drinks. Joe pulls up a fold-
ing chair, so close their knees nearly touch, and they talk about the day.
They are fifty-one. They've been married more than half their lives, and
they sit quietly each night with their son. Jon can hold the bottle by himself, but he doesn't; he grabs his mother's finger and, like his father, he
hangs on.

8 Hello, My Love

In April 1994, shortly after she moved to the United States for her husband's job, Anna began visiting doctors for infertility treatment. She started a diary of the experience, writing in the small, lined pages of a hardcover book a fourth-grade student had given her while she was still teaching in Germany. The cover of the book was fanciful—two snails, a boy and a girl.

Words and impressions of her experience would come to her as she stood in the shower or sculpted. She would write them down whenever she was alone, sometimes in her bedroom, most often as she sat on the back porch of her northern California house overlooking the garden. The diary never left the house. Anna kept it in the top drawer of her dresser, along with laboratory photographs of the embryos she and Stefan had produced, a picture of her mother as a child in Germany, and a photograph of herself with her first niece. She shared the diary with no one. She doubted her husband Stefan knew that it existed. Anna wrote in this small book because she found it was a place to put her anger when she ovulated on a weekend and couldn't undergo artificial insemination because her doctor's office was closed. It gave her a place to grieve over the hurt the world had no idea it was inflicting. Over the years the diary became an outlet, a confidante, a confessor, and, in time, a history. It was a love letter to an unfound child she called "My Love."

(Translated from the German)

Jan. 5, 1995

Hello, My Love,

I don't know if you will ever exist, but if you do, you will be the most loved child on this earth. After a break of one year, we decided yesterday to try again for a victory against our fate which, without mercy, leaves us childless. What for others is the easiest thing in the world is for your dad and me an almost unsolvable problem. My trust in fate has come to an end, and I hope science will have a solution.

Here in the USA everything is different, you can't just see a doctor, you have to go through a certain bureaucratic way. That means before you can go to a specialist you have to ask your primary care physician who wants to run some tests by himself and get some money from the cake. You have to tell your story over and over again. You must undergo tests twice and get examined countless times. But as our doctor so optimistically puts it, "Welcome to California. Within the year you will hold the child of your dreams in your arms."

Maybe this time we will get lucky, and you will, too. Maybe you can be born in this beautiful corner of the world?

April 6, 1995

Hello, My Love,

Five months of bureaucratic and medical work is behind us. The way toward you is not an easy one. But maybe you'll like this month, April, and will be in the mood to get to know the world. Your dad and I are going to try once again for an artificial insemination. One year of "only" love was without result. So sad. With this method there is only a 20 percent success rate—it is not too high—so please, please come into being. Your aunt, my sister, is just creating her second child. It's so unfair.

Your father is still optimistic, but I have difficulties believing you will ever exist, my love.

May 1, 1995

Hello, My Love,

It is so exciting. We just came from the gynecologist, and we got one egg on the right side. (Super!) Is that you? Today is the first of May. Don't you think it's a beautiful day? The sun is shining, the sky laughs. I have decided that the insemination will take place today as late as possible. Then, the egg and the sperm will have enough time to find each other.

My dad (your grandfather) thinks there is still no soul ready to share our life. I think wherever you and your soul are, wherever you wait, today is your day.

May 14, 1995

I see through the window and it rains
drops falling
heavy
out of the gray
sky
like the unfulfilled
longings
of
my soul.

June 12, 1995

Dear Unborn,

Almost two months have gone by, and my continual writing shows the senselessness of our struggle. The saddest thing is that deep down in me I know that you will never exist. Maybe I already wrote this somewhere, I don't know, maybe repeating it makes it more concrete. Nevertheless, in every monthly cycle I have this crazy, unfortunate, fatal, presumptuous hope that it is going to work by itself! It is so senseless. My bleeding body is grieving. In three months I will be thirty-four years old. Every insemination reduces the eggs I have. My mom was thirty-eight when she went into menopause. There is the chance of inheriting the early menopause. By then everything is over.

My girlfriend is expecting her first child. I am so happy not to live near her anymore. I will not, I cannot, have contact with her any longer. . . .

July 20, 1995

We decide to skip the artificial insemination, take our money, and go to a fertility clinic. For me, everything goes too slowly. They require endless tests, mostly from me, some hurtful, some time-consuming. And in the end, you feel really sick, but nobody can see it. In spite of these challenges, we get into the program and off we go.

Anna's medical records: Patient Anna P. is thirty-three years of age and has never been pregnant. She and her husband have been married twelve years. Seven years with no birth control. Hysterosalpingogram suggests total blockage on the left fallopian tube and partial blockage on right. She used an IUD before and may have had a pelvic infection. She has history of elevated prolactin levels and thyroid disease. Sperm counts are normal. This couple has been trying for many years and the X ray has given us a clue that there is a potential problem with the tubes. We're at a crossroads. Either we investigate the cause and try and correct what's mechanically wrong in the pelvis or the other option is to not waste any more time trying to categorize, but go straight to in vitro fertilization.

Sept. 11, 1995, patient comes in for hysteroscopy, direct inspection of the uterus, normal, thyroid palpable. Tests positive for phospholipid antibodies, recommend heparin and aspirin.

September 1995

Oh my God! Had I known! All these medications, all these syringes. I have to give myself shots in the leg and in the tummy.

With every new blood test my medication list gets longer. No wonder I can't get a child of my own. My body is an antibaby machine.

Oct. 10, 1995

The egg retrieval. The doctor is optimistic. I make ten follicles and we get nine eggs.

Oct. 13, 1995

The day of the embryo transfer arrives. The doctor tells me the good news is all nine fertilize. The bad news is they are all poor-quality embryos. The number of cell divisions is low, two and three cells. They like to see four to eight. All are heavily fragmented. I feel once more like a failure. He wants to put all nine eggs back in my uterus. Nine embryos!!! I feel tears rising in my throat. That's terrible. I can barely speak, we drag ourselves into the embryo transfer room taking along the first picture of our nine children. I can't look anyone in the eyes. I just feel miserable. The whole procedure is horrible. I cry silently. Stefan is holding my hand. This should be a joyful moment, a moment of hope of positive thinking, but it is only awful. After one hour we drive home exhausted and unhappy.
    It didn't work.

Anna's medical records, Oct. 23, 1995. Patient notified beta pregnancy test results are negative. Stop all medication. Advised counselor available. Schedule conference with doctor. Expect heavy period in seven to ten days.

Nov. 27, 1995

I don't know where I get the power to try it again. I must be crazy. But my star is rising. New doctor is Dr. Zouves. He finds out that my cervix is not straight and you have to make a little twist to get in the uterus. I begin to trust him.

Christmas 1995

I have to take more medication. Nonetheless, we get fewer eggs. The most depressing news comes, again, just before the embryo transfer. Only two fertilized eggs. Bad quality, too. Dr. Zouves can't explain it. Stefan's sperm seems not to be getting through. So next time, if there is a next time, we'll try ICSI. The egg retrieval seems like an egg competition for big chickens. With envious big ears I overhear the whispering from the neighbors. "Very good! We got twenty or twenty-four or fifteen eggs." I have so little to show after so many drugs. I feel like a failure even in the world of the infertile patient.

Zouves's Notes, Dec. 31, 1995: Eleven eggs retrieved, on the following morning only three of the eleven have fertilized. Two embryos. Note that the number of eggs and sperm is the same as in the previous cycle but there is very poor attachment to eggs. Looks like the sperm is just not attaching. Embyros are only two- to four-celled and heavily fragmented. Possible causes? Stimulation or intrinsic egg problem. Considered lab problem but no other patients exhibit poor-quality embryos that day. His sperm, her egg, or combination? This is definitely a setback.

Stefan recalls:
We have been together a long time, since high school. For a time, she didn't want children, and then, later, she wanted them very badly. She worked on me for a year, and finally, for her birthday, I gave her a pacifier, wrapped in a paper that said, "No comment." At first we tried like all couples, and nothing happened. They checked her blood and ovulation. Then they found her prolactin is a little high, and the doctor said, "This is it. You have to take these pills." But she would take them and it would not do anything. Then they say, "You are the one, your sperms are bad," and that was really miserable and depressing.

    When we arrive in California, the first doctor we see, a primary care doctor, says, "Welcome to California! Within a year you will hold the child of your dreams in your arms." He didn't know anything. In the fertility clinic, the worst part is always the embryo transfer, going in and finding out there were bad eggs and then poor-quality embryos and yet trying to be optimistic about it. The longer it takes, the harder it gets. The time in between gives you the ability to forget about the bad parts. Anna used to say, when the wish for a child is this big, you do whatever you have to do.

Zouves's Notes, May 19, 1996: Plan third cycle. We're going to go with ICSI and assisted hatching. Maxing out protocol, we don't have a stronger stimulation.

June 16, 1996: 8:30 A.M. retrieval. Eleven eggs, she's in average range, we do ICSI, his sperm stays the same, no better or worse, six eggs fertilize and one is abnormal. Four continue to grow three to five cells, divisions are low, quality slightly better but still fragmented.

June 19, 1996: Assisted hatching on four right before transfer. Easy transfer.

June 29: Results negative. NOTE: Anna is young, never pregnant, and not even a nibble, zero implantation. It's a very tough situation. Failed three times with the most aggressive treatment we know.

Stefan remembers:
This last time, we do everything right. We did ICSI, she has the IVIG, all the infusions and the shots. We get four good embryos. We are very optimistic, everything goes well. Because we are in the city, we decide to stop by the clinic. I think I'll just run up and get the results of the blood test so we won't have to wait around all day tomorrow. Inside, I realize at once it's a mistake. Everyone is avoiding my eyes, and it is unbelievable that I have done this.

One should not get the results in person, just for oneself.

June 29, 1996

I said I would wait in the car. My whole body goes rigid and at the same time, I am shaking and trembling, praying. Was this it? The moment I see him coming toward the car I know everything is over. His whole body language, dropped shoulders, walking slowly like under a big weight, tells me. Before he ever reached the car, I began to cry. "No, no, no it's not true." Everything in vain, empty.

At home, after drinking lots of champagne, I told Stefan that I had not the power to try again. I needed time to heal, my body and my soul.

1996–1997

I try to see the future without children. I sit on the stairs staring into our garden, seeing nothing and thinking the same thoughts. Why me? Why me? What did I do wrong?

In this process of my infertility treatment, I have read a lot of books about the subject but always skipped the last depressing chapters like "Coping with Childlessness," and "Childless Life" and "Living Without." Now I find myself reading exactly those chapters. I tell my family and friends that I have given up. I can live without my own child. I enjoy my sculpture class at the college and my nice little adult life.

Taboo: whole sections of kids' items, books, toys, clothes. This is a world I cannot enter. Stefan's best friend has two kids, and I find excuses not to accompany them on outings. I am glad my sister and brother and their kids live far away. I tell my mother on the phone that I can live without knowing who is pregnant again. I pretend there are no children in my world.

Stefan recalls:
Her sculptures are long, willowy figures in wood, bronze, stone. They don't have any eyes or mouths. There's always something missing. And this one is crying, and that one is screaming.

After a year, I say to her, "All right, we have the money. Will it be a baby or a house?"

"Oh my God," she says. "This is a hard decision."

I tell her a baby. A baby will be worth it.

March 17, 1997

I'll do it for Stefan. If we fail, I will survive and survive with the good conscience of knowing I've done everything in my power.

We contact the clinic and sign a three-trial contract for $13,775. The two tries contract for $10,000 would have been more than enough for me. To go back to the clinic after one year was a funny feeling. They greet me like an old friend. Some staff are new, and I want to explain to them that I already know everything they want to explain to me. I see my thick file compared to others and try not to take it too seriously. We're doing this lightly; when Stefan gives me a shot, he calls it baby fertilizer.

Zouves's Notes, March 18, 1997: Anna's case is looking more and more like a tough nut. We check both chromosomes, at this point we're scratching our heads, is there something really rare here that we are missing? An underlying problem? Chromosomal tests are normal. We'll adjust her protocol, start stronger, and drop off as we go.

May 6, 1997

Hello, My Love,

It seems I will never hold you in my arms. Again and again, fate throws pain into my path. I had started taking the Pill when my girlfriend made an appointment for me—without my knowledge—with an acupuncturist. The acupuncturist, Miss J*, doesn't believe in my infertility treatment. She had her own ideas about treatment and tries her best to convince me to stop the Western way. I let her talk and think, Why not let both powers work for you? She tried it with needles, and I had to drink lots of the most horrible-tasting teas. When she heard of my imminent IVF, she suggested enemas. I had never had something like that. Yikes. She said it would heal me from the inside. Maybe it will help. Miss J* says to do it every day (!) until the egg retrieval. The first time was unpleasant. The second time I got cramps and broke out in a cold sweat. Today, day 7, I got these awful cramps. I tell Miss J*, and she begins massaging my tummy. Suddenly she looked alarmed. She pressed and pressed, and it hurt a lot. Then she throws a bombshell and said there is a tumor and I should to go a real doctor to have it checked out. I was just about to start with the main fertility *drug. Hopeless, in tears, I drove home. Since I've always had a nervous stomach, I pray to God it is just stress. Again my body doesn't know whether it's up or down; no wonder I can't get pregnant. The experience with Miss J* was only negative. I won't go there any longer, she scares me. I will get an urgent appointment with a real doctor tomorrow. One night I'm dreaming of my own child, and the next, it's about surviving and always there is a feeling, a lonely fight.*

May 20, 1997

Hello My Love,
Thank God Miss J* was wrong. It seems everything is okay with my stomach, although it is now black and blue because of the heparin shots, what Stefan calls the baby fertilizer. It is supposed to convince you and your five brothers and sisters to stay in place. One Love is all I need and then maybe an adoption? What am I talking about? I'm talking as if you are already a reality. I must have as much faith and hope as possible. You wouldn't believe how superstitious one gets. Around my wrist I wear the old rosary from my birthplace. Every time I take the little silver cross in my palm, it gets warm and I relax. It's my new talisman.

Zouves's Notes, May 21, 1997: 10:30 A.M. transfer. Egg retrieval eight eggs, six fertilize. Grade one embryos are flawless, equal in size and shape and blemish-free. Grade twos are nearly perfect, and grade three are slightly more irregular and fragmented. We end up with three grade twos and three grade threes. One has seven cells. For the first time we're seeing embryos above the four-celled stage on the third day. Still not great but definite improvement. We do assisted hatching on all six, and the transfer is easy. She is on 20 g of IVIG, as well as heparin and aspirin.

May 27, 1997

Katya threw her magic stones (Runen) for me. She got the X, it means a present from God. I produce only six fertilized eggs. But this time one is good and two were okay. During the transfer I hear ocean noises and a seagull cries. I drift off dreaming about little babies. It is a full moon when I get my embryos back. I play solitaire, and the bet was: A baby or not? I won without tricks.

May 28, 1997

In the middle of the night, I wake up all sweaty and think everything is over. My body felt the old familiar emptiness. No promising little pull or pressure, only me, endlessly alone. This morning my breasts no longer feel swollen. Together with the nightly hot flashes, a sure sign the hormones are going into the cellar. Pregnancy, bye bye. Again, there will be no soul for my little embryos. I am so sad. I try to explain it to Stefan, and he says, "Why are you sure?" I cannot explain it. It is a combination of body language and intuition; I cannot explain it. I know if it is not happening this time, it never will happen at all. I am so unbelievably sad.

Zouves's notes, May 31, 1997: Pregnancy test positive. Advised patient, very excited and will come in 6-1 to review. Too excited to even go into instructions.

May 31, 1997

Hello, My Love,

What a pessimistic human being your MOTHER is. On Saturday we got the most important news in our whole life. Your existence. You are there, in me, growing and growing. Your father and I both cried when we heard the news. He ran outside and I followed him and we held each other and tears of joy were streaming down our cheeks. I suddenly feel so precious holding you inside me.

Life gets a meaning.

Zouves's Notes, June 23, 1997: Almost a day to the year from her third negative cycle, ultrasound scan shows that two sacs have implanted, roughly equal in size, the second one a little smaller. Both have heartbeats.

July 9, 1997: The second sac is smaller and has not pro-gressed, no heartbeat. Other one growing very nicely, gone from 6 to 28 millimeters in size. This is the vanishing twin syndrome. It was not for lack of hormonal or immunological support, we think that maybe nature knew there was problem and just switched off growth.

Aug. 1, 1997: Immunophenotype, the natural killer cells were at 22, clearly elevated, normal is 14 so she stays on IVIG and will test her again. Explain that these are the immune sys-tem's defense against infection and foreign tissue but that they can become misdirected and turn against the pregnancy.

Aug. 28, 1997: Natural killer cells at 20 percent. Advise to stay on IVIG and heparin and aspirin. Advise that there is clearly evidence the immune system is still hyperactive and these cells can damage the placenta and after having had one twin vanish I don't know if stopping the medication now could precipitate loss. For safety's sake we should probably just continue.

Sept. 26, 1997: We tested again and natural killer cells up 26 percent. The bigger the baby gets, the more cells are kicking in.

Oct. 3, 1997: She is at eighteen weeks and natural cells had gone up.

Oct. 31, 1997: NK cells same. Tell patient the placenta is get-ting to the size where it should be able to defend itself against these natural killer cells but there is a chance the placenta could be damaged and cause growth reduction in baby. Make this her last IVIG and give doctor recommendation to monitor for intrauterine growth retardation, low amniotic fluid, placental insufficiency, when repeat natural killer cells test in four weeks.

Nov. 24, 1997: Patient at twenty-four weeks and natural killer cells come back at 28 percent. At this point we make a decision to stop, but her doctor is onboard and they're going to have her come in every two weeks for ultrasound and nonstress testing. Placenta is big enough to look after itself. I think we've carried her far enough. Recommend careful surveillance. Most people are done with immunotherapy by the end of twelve weeks. Due date 2-11-98.

Feb. 17, 1998: Delivery. Baby girl, normal vaginal birth 8-14 ounces. Huge! Definitely no growth reduction, I would argue, because of prolonged immunotherapy given positive phospholipids and thyroid antibodies.
CONGRATULATIONS!

Postscript

August 1998

Dear Dr. Zouves and staff,

The first time Caro smiled at me I had to cry tears of joy because for so many years I never thought it would be possible ever to hold my own child. And it's not only the feeling to have one's own child. It's also the feeling to finally belong to the rest of the world, to be normal and whole, like before the whole infertility nightmare started. Would you believe that I would already love to have a brother or sister for her. As if this would be easy (money and body wise). Always thankful,
Stefan and Anna.

Stefan says:
She kept all her unused needles, maybe she'll need them again. She sees it as still her condition. I think you should be happy with your life. I also clearly remember that it wasn't easy to go through the emotional pain, I don't even want to think of going through that again. It can spoil your life.

September 1998

Hello, My Love,

I am so blessed. When you think about it, it's such a low percentage when it works. It's a little miracle that I got you. I am the lucky one. When I look at Caro I see this person, my God this person was inside me and Stefan, always there, but she couldn't exist without all these things. It is so weird, I am so thankful in this case that someone could get her out.

9 An Open Book

*L*ove came late and sat three rows behind her.

Kathryn was almost forty and had all but given up on a long-term, committed relationship since her first marriage ended fourteen years earlier. She had a career as a financial auditor, a beautiful condominium, a new car, and many friends. She'd been taking self-development courses through the Summit Organization, trying to figure out why she hadn't found Mr. Right when, three rows back, she found him.

Paul was an architect. When he bought a three-story 1892 Victorian in San Francisco, it had been condemned for bad plumbing, bad wiring, and no exits. He poured seven years of time and twice the purchase price into the house, bringing luster to the hardwood floors, light in through the bay windows, and voices to the thirty-two-step staircase that reached up to the third floor. He rebuilt several historic buildings around San Francisco and worked on city efforts to preserve and protect others. When his marriage dissolved midlife, he began his own rehab, signing up for self-improvement seminars.

At Summit workshops, participants independently analyze their families, regrets, and goals. By the time Paul and Kathryn met, they knew where they were in life and where they wanted to go. She knew she wanted to get married. He knew he wanted to have children. Within two months of meeting, they were in a scuba-diving class, in Hawaii, in love. Within a year, they were married and living in Paul's renovated Victorian. Within three months of the wedding, they were in a six-week workshop called "The Baby Debate."

Kathryn had never been around children and when she thought about them the first words that came to mind were *responsibility*, *duty*, and *work*. Paul, who had twenty-six nephews and nieces he had spent a lot of time with, answered in one syllable: *joy*. He had an infectious sense of family, pulling Kathryn close to relatives she hadn't seen in years. Paul was a man who took the blood ties between people seriously. When they decided that they wanted a family, she was already forty-one and he was forty-four.

They went straight to a fertility doctor. For the first six months they tried ovulation drugs and carefully timed sex, to no avail. During the next six months they underwent intrauterine insemination. In the midst of all this, Kathryn had three surgeries to diagnose and treat ovarian cysts, and Paul underwent surgery to treat varicocele—varicose veins in the testicles, a condition that warms the scrotum enough to lower sperm count. Tying off or occluding the veins could improve chances for his sperm, but it doesn't work for everyone. In March 1992, more than fourteen months had passed and they were no closer to parenthood. Kathryn's gynecologist referred them to our center.

As they arranged to undergo an in vitro fertilization cycle with one of my old partners, Kathryn wrote in her journal that her dream was "to have a beautiful daughter to share our happiness and joy with. . . . Someone who will share her wisdom, who will truly make a difference in the quality of the world."

On May 17, at her egg retrieval, Kathryn produced eight follicles, and eggs were retrieved from every one. Kathryn and Paul were full of hope when they came in for the transfer. Instead they were escorted into the doctor's office and told there would be no transfer. The news was crushing. None of the eggs had fertilized. When the doctor began describing what they should do on the next cycle, Paul and Kathryn were too stunned to reply. After ten minutes, they got up and left. In a marriage based on open communication and disclosure, they almost never spoke of that day again. It was too saddening.

That spring they went to a symposium sponsored by the national infertility support group RESOLVE, conducted at Mills College in California. Paul was more convinced than ever that he wanted children. Kathryn wasn't sure how she felt after everything they'd been through. Every woman she'd ever talked with had said that motherhood was the best experience she'd had. It wasn't until she heard a forty-something man who'd recently become a father speak that she realized other people also felt ambivalent about this leap.

"I had to go on intellectual faith that all the things friends had been telling me about parenthood were going to be true for me, too," the man said.

When Paul and Kathryn returned home, they called me.

When Kathryn and Paul come into the office June 18, we discover that members of both Paul's family and my family were builders and architects. His father was a first generation Norwegian builder in Minnesota, and mine was a first generation Greek builder and architect in Kimberley, South Africa. Paul became an architect. I considered the field only briefly. My sister is the artist in the family. But I always start my work with patients by asking about their work. One of the joys of my life is the variety and intelligence of the patients I treat.

My work with patients ends in their twelfth week of pregnancy when they go on to their regular doctor. But our working relationship may last years. It may take a couple one month, two years, or five years to have a successful pregnancy. Many couples, like Paul and Kathryn, I get to know well. Others I must get to know within a few weeks, in order to have a relationship in which I can assemble the variables of their case and they can feel comfortable telling me things germane to solving their problem.

Paul and Kathryn and I are all aware that they face significant hurdles. Kathryn is forty-four. We know that, for women her age, the chances of taking home a baby with her own eggs in an in vitro fertilization cycle are only about 2 or 3 percent. I review the fact that Paul's sperm count is still on the low side with very poor motility, and add that I suspect sperm antibodies may also be a factor. We don't really know why the male body begins producing antibodies to attack its own sperm, although it is quite common in men after vasectomy. Other suspected causes include an injury to the testicle or an infection. Paul tests 100 percent positive for sperm antibodies, which means his sperm clump, they stick together. As a result, they can't penetrate the egg. Based on their sperm and egg factors, this couple has six options. They can use donor sperm and try to inseminate Kathryn during a natural cycle, a stimulated cycle, or an in vitro fertilization cycle. They can use donated eggs with either donor sperm or Paul's sperm. A fifth option may be embryo donation. And sixth, they can adopt a baby.

Kathryn and Paul have spent more than $10,000 on fertility treatments already. They begin to consider option six, adoption. In August, they call the Independent Adoption Center, an independent agency that specializes in open adoptions. The amount of disclosure and counseling sessions the agency offers for all parties involved appeals to them. The way Paul and Kathryn see it, it's less likely that a young frightened birth mother will change her mind in the hospital if she's been fully informed and feels comfortable with the adoptive parents beforehand. They also believe that, with an open approach, their child will have fewer questions about his or her origins.

The agency advises Kathryn and Paul to write a letter to a prospective birth mother, keeping in mind the photographs they include are as important as the text. The letter will also go into a collection of 125 letters at the agency. A prospective birth mother reads these letters and chooses a couple she would like to see parent her child.

Their letter is a single sheet of paper with a photo of them, an attractive smiling couple who look to be about forty. Also pictured are Paul pushing a stroller, their cat named Susie Q., and Kathryn baking cookies.

They write:

Dear Birth Mother:

We respect your courage in taking control over the wellbeing of your baby now and for the future. This difficult decision shows your strength of character, values and loving spirit, traits that we admire in people and want in our children. Paul and I hope you will consider us as parents for your baby.

We met at a personal-growth workshop six years ago. Open communication and commitment are critical as the basis of our relationship. We have been married over four years, and our relationship grows stronger every day. In a workshop a year after we were married, Paul and I wrote a mission statement for our lives together, which we would like to share with you.

"To sustain a loving committed relationship through continual personal growth and interdependence . . . and through our joy to be an inspiration to everyone who touches our lives." Becoming parents will provide us an opportunity to bring another dimension to this purpose, living a life even fuller than we do today.

Today is wonderful. We have made our home in a sunny, warm Victorian house with a fluffy little Persian cat named Susie Q. Our home is close to two beautiful parks with wonderful children's playgrounds. Both of us love scenic beauty and the outdoors and enjoy jogging along the Bay paths, hiking in the woods, and skiing at Lake Tahoe. We love to travel and look forward to providing the excitement and wonder of new places to our child. Although our moms and most of our brothers and sisters are not in the Bay area, we share many holidays with them and see them often. We have a large and caring group of close friends, many with children under four. Together they provide us the warmth and support of a truly loving extended family. We are most fortunate, and we dream of sharing this life with a child. Warmly, Kathryn and Paul.

Kathryn and Paul also send the letter to three hundred people in twelve countries. They join a support group with four other couples in Marin County, all waiting to adopt. One year later, everyone in the group is still waiting. Kathryn and Paul have received just one phone call from a prospective birth mother that developed no further.

Feeling like time and their options are quickly passing, they call me back and on February 17, come in to discuss what I meant when I said "embryo donation."

I explain that embryo donation is a new concept for all of us. When couples have completed their families through in vitro fertilization, they have the option of keeping their embryos cryopreserved for future use or disposing of them by having the embryos removed from the culture in which they are stored, which causes the cells to disintegrate and die. A third option we are just beginning to offer these families is the chance to donate their embryos anonymously to another couple. Because the number of embryos donated is small, we can offer them only to couples who have undergone unsuccessful treatment at our center. Kathryn and Paul fit the bill. Embryo donation could be the perfect solution for them.

Ethicists frown upon the deliberate creation of embryos for adoption. And indeed, Kathryn and Paul could "create" their own embryos using a donor egg and donor sperm. But given that these embryos we have at the center already exist, it is good to find a home for them.

Ethically, I believe being born to loving, but unrelated, parents is not harmful to a child. Embryo donation also strikes me as more respectful of embryos that already exist and would otherwise be destroyed.

Paul and Kathryn have begun calling the arrangement we are discussing "embryo adoption," and indeed it is a little like that. They would be adopting an embryo from a couple who would share information about its genetic and medical histories. Many donated embryos result from IVF cycles where donor eggs or donor sperm were used. Counseling is required for all parties. But unlike a classic adoption, there is no home study and no judge.

One of the largest ethical challenges to embryo adoption is disclosure. First, all parties fully discuss the medical, legal, and psychological risks of the immediate procedure and the possible long-term ramifications. What, if anything, will the intended parents tell the child? Many psychologists and adoption specialists say openness will prevent long-term psychological problems in the child and create successful families by making children feel wanted, and not abusing their trust. Yet, many families struggle with how, and how much, to tell.

When Paul and Kathryn call, we are in the midst of writing our embryo adoption protocol, and so far, there are no embryos available. Many couples who have already conceived and delivered a baby decline to donate their remaining embryos, saying they don't want a full genetic sibling to their child out there in the world. I ask Kathryn and Paul to telephone the center every three months to see if any embryos become available for adoption.

Then, in late October, a married couple who had in vitro fertilization and delivered twins volunteers to donate eight frozen embryos. They were created with the wife's eggs and donor sperm. Kathryn and Paul are first on the donation list. They balk at the paperwork that calls for complete anonymity and confidentiality. They want there to at least be the means to exchange information someday if it is amenable to both parties. Being an in vitro fertilization program and not a formal adoption agency, we opt for anonymous embryo adoption as our standard procedure.

"We really want to leave the door open to more openness," Kathryn says as we meet to discuss the arrangement. This couple's attempts to adopt a child have convinced them that openness is best for everyone.

"It's for the children, not for us. There is nothing shameful about this, so why have all this secrecy? In this process, I'll be the birth mother, but I want my baby to know he or she could have a sibling out there."

Kathryn remembers a passage she read about egg donation, that the process creates not just a newborn, but a whole person who in time will become a teenager, a parent, and a grandparent. Kathryn and Paul see the child as a person who has the right to be loved, safe, and secure, and to know his personal history.

Ethicist David Thomasma calls what Kathryn and Paul are doing "imaginative reasoning," the kind of thinking that he feels we are called to do when we are involved in reproductive technologies. We cannot possibly foresee all the consequences of embryo donation, for instance; but we have a responsibility to try to foresee as much as we can. This is a difficult task. Thomasma says that whenever we intervene in a natural process, we have a responsibility to consider the consequences of that intervention, not only on a woman's health, but on the family structure and perhaps our very society. Whether people agree with Kathryn and Paul's call to openness, one must appreciate their concern and vision.

At last, responding to Kathryn and Paul's plea, the donating couple agrees to the possibility of being contacted someday through an exchange of mail through the center. We proceed to collect and forward the medical histories of both the egg and sperm provider. We also test again for infectious diseases, and counsel all parties involved. Once counseling is completed in late October, I prescribe Kathryn's medications to prepare her body to carry a pregnancy, just as we would if she were receiving donated eggs. She takes natural estrogen and progesterone to thicken the lining of her uterus.

Kathryn prepares physically, emotionally, and spiritually for the cycle. She writes in her journal, "I awoke this morning thinking of my unborn child. Let him (or her) know how loved and wanted he is, not just by Paul and me but by the giving and selflessness of the couple releasing the embryos. People helping other people making dreams come true. What a heart this child of ours will have, with such a lovely beginning. We are all related. Truly."

On November 16, eight embryos are removed from a liquid nitrogen tank, thawed in a water bath, and rehydrated. Children have been born from cryopreserved embryos since 1984.

Embryos frozen at the four- to eight-cell stage have the advantage that, even if a cell or two or five is lost in process, the embryo can still survive the thaw, implant, and grow into a healthy baby. Yet, anywhere from 10 to 30 percent of the embryos do not survive the thaw. They also implant at about half the rate that fresh embryos do. Studies have shown that the babies born from frozen embryos are as healthy and whole as those born through other types of assisted reproduction. A frozen embryo transfer is much less demanding and expensive since it involves only the end of the in vitro fertilization cycle, the transfer. Six of the eight embryos donated to Paul and Kathryn survive, and the following morning we agree to transfer all six.

At Thanksgiving dinner with relatives the same week, Kathryn skips the wine. The next afternoon, the nurse telephones to say her pregnancy test is negative. It is another disappointment. By this time, there is a list of twenty to thirty families on the waiting list to adopt donated embryos, and Kathryn and Paul now must move from first to last on the list. It seems hopeless. They consider international adoption from the former Soviet Union, but are so frustrated by the adoption agency, they back off. As they have every month since 1990, they sit back and wait.

Two days before Valentine's Day, the telephone rings in their Victorian house. It's "Lisa," a pregnant nineteen-year-old woman calling. She has read their "Dear Birth Mother" letter and wants to meet to discuss giving up her baby. Kathryn and Paul both get on the telephone. They talk for nearly an hour and arrange to meet her for coffee the following Sunday. Lisa never shows up. She never calls back. The adoption agency has never heard of her.

"We go from one roller coaster to the next," Kathryn writes in her journal. "Never in control."

On April 29, my staff notifies Kathryn and Paul that they have come to the top of the list again and that another couple has agreed to donate their stored embryos. Kathryn begins twice-weekly shots of estrogen on May 23.

Seven days later, "Lisa" the birth mother who telephoned them before, telephones again. They haven't heard from her in three months. She is in California, five months' pregnant, and wants to talk again. Kathryn and Paul agree to meet her, and when they hang up the telephone, they stare at each other helplessly. After five years of trying to have a baby with no luck, in a single week the possibility of two children is within their grasp. But after everything they have been through, the chance of either coming to fruition seems remote.

"The in vitro hasn't worked before, and this one may not work, especially with my age," Kathryn says. "Lisa might change her mind. I don't know; both are long shots."

"We want more than one child anyway," Paul says. "Let's see what happens."

They agree at least to meet Lisa and arrange to pick her up at her grandparents' house. When the pregnant young woman opens the door, Paul about falls across the threshold. She looks just like his nieces. The three-year-old boy holding her leg is her son, doe-eyed beautiful.

"I'm thinking she's the birth mother from heaven," Paul remembers. The next few hours are like those sweet, short days just after you fall in love. When all the world and everybody in it looks wonderful. The baby Lisa is carrying is her third unplanned pregnancy, she explains. A couple in the Bay area has already adopted her second child, a daughter, and her grandparents are helping her raise her first, the little boy. The children have different birth fathers.

Kathryn and Paul and Lisa then drive to a café, eat sandwiches, and talk for two hours. Kathryn and Paul are praying that she likes them. They don't want to scare Lisa off by telling her she has contacted them in the middle of an in vitro fertilization cycle. They also want to be fair and honest. They decide they'll tell her as soon as they know if the cycle works.

Six days later Kathryn comes into the clinic for the embryo transfer. The donors are a forty-something couple who used an egg donor, a pre-med student from Berkeley whose heritage is Norwegian. The night before the transfer, Paul opens a bottle of Dom Perignon. As they share this bottle of celebration and hope, they admit they are scared that the in vitro process won't work and a little scared that it will. They hadn't deliberately pursued an instant family, yet, before them are two possible paths to parenthood. They are aware of the responsibility and commitment that more than one child requires, and, at the same time, they are terrified that both attempts will end in disappointment. They don't know how they'll survive another failure. That night they raise a toast to all the people helping them start their family and, lastly, to each of their mothers.

"Skol," he says, for luck.

"Skol."

"I love this man," Kathryn writes in her journal that evening. "It is past time he has his own children to grow up and bless the world."

The next morning, I transfer six thawed and growing embryos. Kathryn has been taking progesterone and estrogen to prepare her uterus for the pregnancy. Since the first failed transfer, she has tested positive for phospholipid antibodies, which means that she may have trouble getting an embryo to implant and grow. So she's been taking twice-daily shots of heparin and a baby aspirin a day to combat that. The transfer is completed successfully. Now we wait.

Within five days, Kathryn says she *feels* pregnant. On June 19, tests confirm that she is. On July 7, I have the joy of pointing out on the ultrasound a single uterine pregnancy, with a clear fetal pole and strong heartbeat. They are thrilled.

For years, people have believed there is a direct connection between deciding to adopt and getting pregnant, as though one event precipitates the other. We know from studies that this observation is mostly anecdotal and not borne out by statistics. A certain number of people will conceive spontaneously and would have regardless of taking steps toward adoption. But the simultaneous timing of this adoption and conception never ceases to amaze me.

Kathryn lies awake half the night worrying about what she will tell Lisa. She opts for the truth: They've spent almost six years trying every means to have a family, and now that they have found their perfect adoptive birth mother, they're pregnant.

"Wow," Lisa says when she hears their news. Instead of backing off, the birth mother warms to the idea that the baby will have a brother or sister. She'd like to proceed with the adoption. Kathryn and Paul can't believe it. The family they've dreamed of is moving within their reach.

Many adoption professionals are concerned about the adoption of two unrelated children within months or weeks of each other. Some say that "artificial twinning" can have some negative long-term effects on a child's sense of self; they also agree that the success depends on how supportive the relationships are between the parents and each child.

Openness and awareness are key, the three adults learn when they proceed to the adoption agency, where they begin a series of counseling sessions and agreements on how open their relationship will be, what Kathryn and Paul should do at the hospital, and who will arrange contact between the two families.

Day after day, the babies inside the two women grow. Kathryn is worried Lisa will change her mind.

Lisa never wavers.

Postscript

Kathryn never had any illusions that pregnancy would be wonderful or empowering. So when it was both, it surprised her. Suddenly the body shape that she'd fought her whole life was exactly right, the round hips, thighs, and breasts that she had bemoaned for years were now just perfect. She felt healthy and strong, with no hint of complications. What frightened her at this point wasn't her own pregnancy, but Lisa's. She discovered that Lisa had not been honest about her prenatal care. At almost eight months' pregnant, Lisa had never seen a doctor.

Kathryn quickly began arranging appointments and meeting Lisa at the doctor's office to ensure she'd show up. She did.

Lisa delivered on October 7, a perfect baby girl they named Marie. Paul held the infant while Kathryn, four months' pregnant, cut the umbilical cord.

Soon Kathryn was climbing those steep old Victorian stairs with a newborn infant in her arms and her forty-seven-year-old body carrying the couple's second child.

Two months before her due date, Kathryn's doctor began closely monitoring her high-risk pregnancy, and within four weeks she developed preeclampsia. Her ankles swelled as she retained fluid, and her blood pressure rose dangerously. Her water broke three weeks early, and she delivered a five pound, thirteen ounce girl, Elizabeth. The baby was so thin that she reminded Paul of a wizened old woman. Kathryn believed the early delivery, her own age (almost forty-eight), and less-than-lush uterine lining were responsible, but I believe that the blood pressure played a part. However, the baby was healthy and after a few weeks of breast-feeding, she plumped right up.

In June, Lisa signed the final documents and a California judge formalized Kathryn and Paul's adoption of baby Marie. The birth father had, through the mail, agreed to terminate his rights. Nonetheless, Kathryn sent him a photo of the child he had fathered, along with their address, in case he ever wanted to contact them or the little girl. She received no response. She and Paul and their two babies continued to see Lisa occasionally. They also contacted the family that had adopted Lisa's second daughter to inform them of a new genetic half-sister. Eventually both sets of adoptive parents and Lisa and her son met in a San Francisco park for a picnic. Since then, Kathryn and Paul have continued to see Lisa and her son several times a year, usually around holidays and birthdays. They have also become quite close with the family that adopted Lisa's second child.

When Elizabeth was nearly a year old, Kathryn contacted our center saying she wanted to contact the family that donated her embryos. She said that, if her daughter had a full genetic sibling somewhere, she wanted to give both children the chance to meet someday. She didn't think that decision should be made solely by the adults who brought the children into the world. We agreed at least to forward Kathryn's letter. Five months later, a letter came back.

Kathryn and Paul opened it and read it together. It was from the donating couple, typewritten on elegant stationery, informative but reserved. They admitted feeling shocked by the contact and a little hesitant. They were worried the exchange of information may open a Pandora's box. Nonetheless, they disclosed that there was indeed a sibling, a full genetic brother, to Elizabeth. He was healthy and beautiful, as the enclosed pictures showed.

The couple wrote that they had lost three babies to miscarriage and stillbirth before seeking in vitro fertilization using donor eggs. When they finally conceived and delivered their son, he was perfect. But the pregnancy was so difficult, it was clear the wife could never carry a child again. They called their son a "miracle" and said that, in the days after his birth, they felt such joy there was no way they could not give that opportunity to someone else and so agreed to donate the embryos.

But they asked Kathryn and Paul for complete discretion. No one in their family knew of their experience except the people who would become the boy's legal guardians if anything happened to them. They wrote to tell Kathryn and Paul that they would share their letter with the intended guardians. Their fear was that their son would learn the circumstances of his conception through someone other than them. So they asked that no contact be made until he was an adult, and that included any contact from a genetic sibling. They would, however, accept another letter at any time. Kathryn was thrilled and satisfied with this response.

The couples have no plans to meet. Kathryn wishes they knew the woman who donated her eggs that became Elizabeth.

"My concern is for my daughter," Kathryn said. "I wrote to the donating couple because I want to someday face my daughter and tell her that I did everything that I could do to find her sibling."

Although they want to know of their existence, Kathryn and Paul do not consider any of the other genetic siblings to be Elizabeth's brother or sister. To them, brothers and sisters are members of the same family, living, loving, growing together day by day. The only sister their daughter has, as far as they're concerned, is the one who shares her bathtub, Marie. Elizabeth is a coordinated, athletic, and very focused child. Marie is talkative and a bit of a butterfly, always zipping around. They are dark and light, opposites, coincidentally, just like their parents. Kathryn and Paul celebrate this unique relationship with a "Family Days" celebration every June 9 and 10, the day one daughter was conceived in vitro and another was legally adopted. "Our dreams have been met beyond all our hopes," Kathryn said. "I'm very proud of how we've put our family together."

10 Bittersweet

"Hey, Mom, the Shot Lady is here."

At seven each night, Kelly, the "Shot Lady," pulled into her neighbor Barbara's West Coast suburban driveway to get her shot of fertility medicine. Barbara was a registered nurse, the mother of two boys, and a friend since childhood. The two women would say hello, then proceed to the bedroom where Barbara would break open a glass ampule of white powder. She would dilute the powdered fertility drugs with water, draw the fluid into a syringe, and inject the needle deep into the muscle of Kelly's buttock. Barbara was always cheerful and efficient, something Kelly's husband, in the face of shots, was not.

The 7 P.M. shot was an act of friendship between women. In friendships, Kelly excelled. She understood women, liked women, and had dozens of women friends. She had girlfriends she made in grade school and kept through her twentieth high school reunion. Once a year, she and her girlfriends went to Lake Tahoe or San Diego, ate indulgently, and stayed up half the night. Kelly loved long phone conversations and hair toys, what she called "girl stuff."

Kelly was married to Mark, and even that was a sweet story of friendship. Their fathers had met forty years earlier when they served together in a mounted U.S. Army regiment in Berlin in 1946. Nearly four decades later, Kelly's father, a retired military officer, announced that he was going to visit his old army buddy who had a ranch in the Southwest. Kelly, who was working as a legal secretary, decided to tag along. The buddy's son, Mark, happened to be home from graduate school. Within five minutes of meeting him, Kelly knew as well as she'd known anything that he was The One.

Three weeks later Mark crossed two states to see Kelly. They went to the wine country, to barbecues, to dinner with friends, drunk on the discovery of how much they had in common: how strictly they were raised; how much they respected authority; how much, with their thin, dark, good looks, they were alike. People who saw the couple thought they were brother and sister. Kelly and Mark wrote each other every day and talked on the telephone every night. They married at the ranch the summer of 1990. She was thirty-three; he was thirty-two.

A year later, they threw away their birth control. They wanted children because they loved their parents, they loved being part of a family, and they wanted to create more of a family than just the two of them. They wanted a daughter and chose her name before they were even married—Natalie. Mark wanted a girl because he'd grown up in a family of boys. To him, Kelly was the ultimate girl. Kelly used to joke that she couldn't go camping because there was no place to plug in her hair dryer. She had kept all her Barbies. To Mark, her femininity was an exotic break from the past. He loved it and wanted more of it. They both dreamed of a little girl.

Kelly wasn't a superstitious woman, but she had once wondered aloud to her best friend whether she'd have trouble getting pregnant. Mark figured it would happen the first time they had unprotected sex. It didn't.

After eighteen months of trying to conceive, Kelly went to her ob/gyn, who ran initial tests, found a fibroid tumor, and removed it. Around them, friends, co-workers, and even high school girls in the neighborhood were having sex and getting pregnant—a consequence Kelly found increasingly amazing and unattainable. Sex had become clinical and mechanical, the result of possible ovulation and not because she was falling into bed with the husband she loved so much.

By July 1993, Kelly's doctor was recommending she visit our fertility center. Which is how Kelly came to be known in neighborhood lore as the Shot Lady.

. . .

I first meet Kelly as the doctor who is performing her hysteroscopy. Before Kelly and Mark can begin an in vitro fertilization cycle, they must undergo a series of tests, including this direct examination of the uterus.

Looking through the long, thin telescope into the uterus, I see a problem is obvious on Kelly's right side near the fallopian tube. A fibroid mass in the muscular wall of her uterus is protruding into the uterine cavity. In the year since her fibroid surgery, a new fibroid has grown along with another smaller one. Compared to the smooth pink muscle of the uterus, a fibroid looks like a whirl of lightly colored fibrous tissue, layers of white and pink. It's tough tissue, some can even calcify and become hard. Kelly's fibroids appear to be growing within the uterine muscle.

Unless they are very large, most fibroids are harmless. Women may go years without even knowing they exist. But that may change with pregnancy or fertility treatment, and thus affect how we treat certain patients, I tell Kelly. When we stimulate a woman's ovaries during an in vitro fertilization cycle, we intentionally boost the estrogen in her blood to four or five times its normal level. The problem is that almost half of all fibroids grow in response to estrogen. So while we're preparing a woman's uterus to receive an embryo, we may inadvertently be stimulating her fibroids to grow as well.

If Kelly's fibroids were both outside her uterus, I would just leave them alone. But the larger one is protruding into the cavity, and it is larger than five centimeters in diameter. Anything that large can prevent pregnancy by behaving like an intrauterine contraceptive device (IUD) or foreign body in the uterus. A large fibroid can also interfere with embryo implantation. An embryo might implant right on the surface of the fibroid and then wither because there is no good blood supply to the uterine lining at that site. If the pregnancy continues, fibroids can grow along with the baby, causing pain, miscarriage, or premature birth.

What causes fibroids? Kelly asks. If I knew, I'd be a prize winner, I tell her. I do know that one in four women develops fibroids at some time and that they may be more common in African-American and Asian women. But no one has yet discovered why fibroids grow in some women and not in others. I do know Kelly's fibroids have to come out.

They can be removed by laparoscopy allowing her to get back on her feet in two to seven days. I tell her it will be at least eight weeks, though, before she is recovered enough for an in vitro fertilization cycle.

In the operative laparoscopy, I insert a laparoscope through an incision near her navel in order to see the pelvic organs. Then I make three small incisions in a semicircle around her bikini line to insert a series of grasping and cutting tools. Kelly's fibroid is located in such a spot that I'll have to cut all the way through to the uterine cavity, remove the fibroid, and then repair the incision, starting with the deepest layer and stitching my way out. The biggest challenge in a surgery like this is to remove the tissue from the abdomen through the narrow plastic tube and then repair the incision in the uterus. The surgery goes well.

Twelve weeks later, Kelly is fit, feeling good, and ready to begin the IVF cycle. She undergoes the shots, responds well to the drugs, and the retrieval goes well. But on the ultrasound monitor, her lining is measuring thinner than I'd like to see. The ten embryos that resulted from mixing Kelly's eggs and Mark's sperm are heavily fragmented and irregular in shape. On the basis of what I know at this time, I tell Kelly we need to transfer all of them to have any chance of success. The couple agrees and we proceed.

Ten days later, on the day of the pregnancy test, Kelly leaves work early; Mark is already home when she arrives. They sit together on the couch, and she calls the center. The last thing she says before dialing is, "I don't feel pregnant."

She isn't.

We all knew the embryos were not ideal, but this news is still painfully final. Kelly's family comes to visit over the Christmas holidays, helping to provide the distraction and space the couple needs to recover. In February 1994 Mark and Kelly come back to visit me. On the basis of the failed cycle, I'm going to try to increase her estrogen level before the retrieval by adding a suppository, hoping to pump up her lining to improve the chances of implantation. I'm also increasing the fertility drugs in the hope of retrieving a few additional eggs. Mark and Kelly are onboard, eager to start the cycle. The retrieval and subsequent transfer go like clockwork.

This time when they call for the results of the pregnancy test, the nurse says, "Congratulations." Kelly hangs up and immediately calls her best girlfriend, who'd been waiting to hear any news. The couple calls their parents; they count the weeks on the calendar and estimate they'll have an autumn baby. It is glorious news, for nine glorious days. Then, Kelly starts to bleed. Had she not known that she was pregnant, she would have thought she was starting her period. The flow is that frank and that final. By the time she gets to the center, the pregnancy hormone in her blood has already disappeared. Kelly and Mark lay in bed that night wrapped in each other's arms, in grief.

Why did the pregnancy disappear? I am sitting at my desk, Kelly's file open, searching. What did we know about her history, her cycle, his sperm, the stimulation, the egg retrieval? I look at the files of other patients transferred that same week to see if there was some common thread related to the laboratory. There isn't. So, I'm asking, what can we change? Kelly's lining was thinner than I had hoped on the second cycle, despite adding the estrogen. In two cycles, we've transferred a total of twenty-three embryos and had only a fleeting positive test. Everything went as well as we planned, and yet it still didn't work. The couple lives near me, and, as I pass their street driving home, I wonder how they're holding up.

When they come in a few weeks later, I tell Kelly and Mark that we have reached a critical point. We are pushing every button we can. On the basis of her two failures, I have to tell this couple that there is now only about a 15 percent chance that they will take home a baby if they try a third time. That means there is a more than 80 percent chance that they won't. Kelly and Mark want a baby as badly as anyone I've met. This ride has been devastating for them. They have a certain faith in the world, that if you do the right thing and are good people, life pretty much happens as expected. This experience has shaken that foundation.

I think the best thing for Kelly and Mark is for them to take some time to decide whether they should stop treatment and perhaps consider adopting or living child-free. I'd like to work with them again, but I'm not going to give them false hope.

If they still want to keep going, there is one approach we haven't yet tried that might help. I tell them about gestational surrogacy. If we fertilize Kelly's eggs with Mark's sperm and transfer the resulting embryos into a surrogate, it just might get around whatever implantation and rejection factor we seem to be up against. A surrogate would allow them to have their own genetic child. But it would also mean Kelly would have to give up the experience of carrying and delivering that child. This is a terribly difficult conversation to have, and I can see the effect of my words on both of them. But Kelly and Mark need to know exactly what their chances are. The decisions that face us today have physical, emotional, and financial consequences that will affect the rest of their lives. I give them a list of agencies they can contact about recruiting a surrogate and learning the logistics of the procedure. I also set up a meeting for them to speak to our in-house psychologist, Shelly Tarnoff.

Mark and Kelly drag themselves home. Kelly calls the surrogacy center to schedule an interview. After the visit, Kelly is still interested. But the encounter leaves Mark cold.

As far as Mark is concerned, circumstances already seem beyond their control, and surrogacy feels like complete surrender. How do they know the surrogate is taking care of herself or their baby? The whole arrangement feels strange to him, and the cost is downright staggering. By the time they pay the agency, the surrogate's fee, her medical insurance, and travel, it will be at least $40,000. That's barring any complications such as providing the surrogate with a nurse or housekeeper should bedrest be required. No way, he says.

They have a good marriage. They have good jobs. Mark works for an oil company doing exploration; Kelly is a legal secretary. Perhaps their life would not be an absolute void if they didn't have kids, Kelly says quietly. Maybe they aren't meant to be parents. Maybe they're going to the wrong doctor. She decides to contact another in vitro fertilization clinic nearby for a second opinion and arranges to have her records from our office copied and sent. In a telephone consultation, the physician agrees with my approach and doesn't have anything different to propose.

Kelly calls me back to say she and Mark have reached a decision. They have just enough money and just enough grit to try getting pregnant one more time. If it fails, she says, at least she will die knowing she did everything humanly possible to have a child. She'll have grief but not regret. The 85 percent chance of failure I quoted them, at this point, disappears. I tell her I'll support them 100 percent. We are going to do everything in our power to help them take home a baby.

For the third time, her neighbor, Barbara, volunteers to be available every night at 7 P.M. The Shot Lady arrives on schedule every night. Kelly is stronger than the nurse would have ever suspected.

Kelly's cycle goes well, and, at the end, we have eight embryos available. Once again, the embryo quality is less than average, and her uterine lining is still not perfect. At this point, sometimes the only variable we can manipulate is the number of embryos for the transfer. Sometimes that's exactly what it takes. But it also increases the risk of a major multiple that would necessitate selective reduction. We need to be aggressive, and they need to understand the possibility they may get three or more. Mark and Kelly are somber, but they agree that they can reduce.

Mark joins his wife for their third transfer, and they're a little rueful that they are so experienced. At the center, they know exactly which procedure room to enter and what to do. They greet every staff member by name.

"We've become old hands," Mark says, squeezing his wife's hand.

Every cycle builds to the embryo transfer, all the shots, schedules, ultrasound scans, and laboratory preparation. Kelly thinks their entire past has come to this critical point as well. Their image of themselves, their view of the future, their dream of having children have all converged. Either they'll be parents in the next ten days or they won't be. This is it.

Kelly feels a strange calm. At least after this, she will know that they have done everything they could to have a child, she told me. There will be no second-guessing, no doubt that they could have done more. Already, in her mind, she's moving on.

Ten days later, Kelly is at home in the kitchen ironing when the telephone rings.

"I'm pregnant?" she says into the telephone. Mark hears the conversation from the back bedroom and comes out. When she hangs up, he puts his arms around her without a word and they stand for a moment, not saying anything. Then Kelly goes back to ironing and Mark to his work in the other room. Perhaps they sense, even then, that there will be hurdles. Nothing has come to them, so far, without a price.

Every morning, Kelly takes the bus to work, bumping into the city to her office building. One day as she is riding along she is swamped with nausea and has to hurry out of the rear door of the bus to look for a bathroom. She just makes it outside when she vomits on the sidewalk in front of a bank. All over her shoes and skirt. She is mortified. No one on the street will meet her eyes. Morning sickness.

Kelly stops taking the bus. The ferry ride is smoother, but she still has morning sickness. When she is six weeks along, she wakes up early one Sunday morning in late July 1994. She's thinking of her best friend's wedding, scheduled for August 3 in Washington, and her role as matron of honor. As she gets out of bed, she realizes there is blood on her pajamas. She is bleeding. She lies back down immediately, and the sorrow comes on like cramps. It is just after dawn, and she and Mark watch the clock until 7:30 A.M. They could have reached the doctor on call, but decided to wait until our office opens. I'm so glad I'm the doctor working that day. As I arrive at my desk, the call is waiting on hold, and I tell Mark to bring Kelly into the office immediately. She is already on the maximum amount of hormones to support the pregnancy. If she is miscarrying, there is nothing I can do to stop it. But I can give her a blood test and an ultrasound scan, relieving them, at least, of the burden of waiting. Mark later said Kelly wept the entire drive across the Golden Gate Bridge to San Francisco.

I call them right into the examining room. Kelly is pale, almost ashen; Mark is haggard. She is afraid to look at the ultrasound monitor and stares, unseeing, at the ceiling. There is one, two, three—three gestational sacs in the uterus, I say. And one clear heartbeat. I can see a heartbeat.

A single tear fills Kelly's eye and trickles slowly down her face into her hair. It is the last thing she expected.

She is so happy that she hardly protests when I tell her she is not going to the wedding. I'm sorry. I know she has the dress and the tickets and the plans, but I don't want her on a long flight or in stressful situations, hustling through airports or carrying luggage. I want Kelly in bed, taking it easy. I fill out medical emergency verification forms so they can claim a refund on their airline tickets. The couple spend hours on the telephone that afternoon explaining this last-minute change in plans to Kelly's friend.

At almost ten weeks, she starts to bleed again, this time heavily. When she comes in for the ultrasound that I've ordered, she is still shaken and subdued when I show her that the pregnancy is still going strong. The three gestational sacs she is carrying are all still there and are growing. Each has a heartbeat now. In some cases, nature somehow selects the healthiest embryo and allows the smaller, or abnormal, gestational sac to disappear, usually by the tenth week. But not this time. It is obvious to all of us that Kelly is carrying three babies.

Irony is everywhere for the fertility patient. It's apparent in the fact that nearly 1 million teenagers get pregnant each year without thought, while 6 million adults seek treatment for infertility. It's one of the few arenas in life where age and wisdom work against you. It's also where sometimes the results of the technology available to help create life forces one to consider ending a life. After years of trying, Kelly and Mark have gone from having no babies to having too many. It is a nightmare. The joy they should be feeling at this moment, the glorious anticipation of having the family of their dreams, is shadowed by the reality and risk of three babies.

Selective reduction is the medical term for the termination of one or more of the fetuses early in a major multiple pregnancy. I raise the issue from the first time I consult with a couple considering in vitro fertilization. Because of the need, at this time, to transfer multiple embryos, there is for some patients a risk of a major multiple. In each in vitro cycle in our clinic where the egg provider is less than forty, there is a 6 percent chance of three or more embryos implanting. The problem is that the human body is simply not meant to carry three or more babies. A multiple pregnancy puts the mother and all of the children at risk. That is why before treatment ever begins I need to find out whether a couple has thought about selective reduction and whether it is something they can do. I raise the issue again when they come in for the cycle and then again when we plan the number of embryos to transfer.

If people have a religious, moral, or ethical objection to abortion, it's a quick discussion. In fact, it's not even a discussion. I tell them I will transfer only as many embryos as they are willing to deliver and raise. Many people with strong antiabortion feelings don't even pursue in vitro fertilization because it involves multiple sperm, multiple eggs, and multiple embryos with inevitable losses or selection at each level. By some people's definition, life begins with the sperm and egg. For others, it begins with fertilization, for others with the formation of embryos, and for others, when there is sensation in the uterus. Everyone has a different take on when life begins. I try to respect them all.

Now, in 1999, a new culture medium helps us avoid this dilemma by allowing us to grow the embryos in the laboratory to the blastocyst or twenty- to one-hundred-cell stage. Embryos at this stage of development are far more robust and likely to survive and implant. Which is why we can transfer just one or, at the most, two, eliminating the risk of triplets or quadruplets. But this is 1994.

My whole purpose here, the whole reason I got into this field, is to help create life, not destroy it. Everyone who faces selective reduction has a problem with it. From the beginning, Kelly and Mark have been very clear. They feel they could not physically carry or raise more than two babies. But now the discussion of the general and abstract has become personal and specific. No one, however educated or informed, is totally prepared. We talk and talk to couples about the need to consider reducing, but it's like saying to someone, "How do you think you're going to feel if we have to amputate your leg?" It hits you only when the surgeon is about to begin. I think that's the way that we as humans protect ourselves from the emotional and physical traumas of life. Some people will call it denial, but it's also a protective mechanism. Intellectually, we can prepare for an abortion if it means saving the lives of two babies. Emotionally, we come undone. The toughest decision is not to reduce from five to two. The toughest and most common decision patients have to make is between two and three. If you're looking at three babies, do you always reduce? Not always. Many of my patients have elected to have triplets, and they would never utter a word of regret. Medical science has vastly improved the chances and outlooks for these children. But stepping back from emotions and looking at a multiple pregnancy from a purely medical point of view, there is still a line in the sand between two and three. Triplets are born an average of nine weeks earlier than singletons. They die at nineteen times the rate of singletons. Babies born before thirty-four weeks lack surfactant, a chemical that enables the lungs to inflate. As a result, respiratory distress syndrome is the leading cause of death of such premature babies. Preemies also are likely to lack the ability to suck and swallow. A premature infant's brain has a delicate vascular system that may bleed, causing severe neurological damage.

From a sociological and psychiatric point of view, there is also a dramatic difference between two and three children. The happy and media-glorified births of five and six and seven babies do little to show the burden and risk of carrying multiple babies. They never do stories on the triplets lost at twenty weeks, or the severe disabilities that premature birth can cause. You never see the family breaking up on television, but I saw it every day in the neonatal intensive care unit when I worked delivering high-risk pregnancies in British Columbia. To keep three or more children is to risk the health of the children and mother.

Dr. William Andereck, a physician at California Pacific Medical Center and chairman of our ethics committee, calls this reality the gray zone. Andereck says that most laypeople see medical care in terms of black and white. The operation cures you or it kills you, you are sick or you get well, you live or you die. Nobody sees the gray zone, in which people have strokes and live for months, unable to speak or move until they finally succumb. Multiples are squarely in this gray zone. The choice to have three or more babies includes life with that many children. The choice to reduce includes living with that decision, as well. So does this mean that we should limit the number of embryos transferred in order to avoid such a choice? Andereck and I agree that decision must remain between well-counseled patients and their doctors, and not made by a government board or an agency that picks a number that sounds right to them.

Mark and Kelly are in the gray zone. They have become so battle-weary that when they look at the statistics surrounding triplets, they don't wonder if they'll fall under the "worst-case scenarios." They know they will. Kelly feels she has managed to be in every bad-luck category that there is. She is sure this will be no exception. The couple decides that if they are going through the trauma and grief of a reduction, they want to minimize the chance of anything else going wrong. They find a physicians' group that performs genetic testing and reduction. This group of perinatologists specializes in high-risk pregnancy and follows cases from earliest diagnosis through delivery. But they also specialize in genetic counseling and the decisions people must make after an abnormal amniocentesis result. Mark and Kelly decide to test the two fetuses in the uterus that are in the best position to survive.

We know that whenever there are multiples, one of the embryos may not have as optimal a place in the uterus to implant and develop. There is usually one embryo that is significantly smaller because of an abnormality or because it is in a poorer position to survive. That would be the one most likely to be reduced. In the event that all the fetuses and sacs are the same size and appear normal, the decision is to choose the one that is high in the uterus and can usually be reached safely. The physician doing the procedure avoids those around the cervix to avoid trauma to the cervix and the risk of infection.

Mark and Kelly arrange to undergo chorionic villus sampling to find any chromosomal abnormalities in either embryo. Kelly undergoes the test on the two gestational sacs that are to remain. Kelly is almost thirty-eight, and her chances of chromosomal defects are greater than they would have been even three years earlier. This knowledge weighs heavily on the couple. It was a long, dark week waiting for the results from the laboratory. They have scheduled the reduction for a Tuesday morning. The day before they still had no results. Finally, at 5 p.m., Kelly enters an empty office at work and telephones the doctors. A genetic counselor immediately gets on the line.

One baby is fine, the counselor says. The other is not. It's a girl, and tests indicate a high likelihood of Turner's syndrome, a chromosomal disorder in which the child never develops secondary sexual characteristics and has possible learning disabilities. The baby could have all of those conditions, could have a few, could have none; there is no way to know until birth. When Kelly hangs up the telephone, she is in a near hysterical state. By the time Mark meets her at the house, she is screaming.

As much as they wanted a girl, in a million years they didn't expect that kind of news. The next morning Kelly and Mark drive south to meet the genetic counselor and physician; they discuss their situation for nearly an hour. They decide not to test the third fetus at that point but will undergo amniocentesis at fifteen weeks. They plan to reduce the fetus with the abnormal test result.

On top of all the stress in deciding to reduce, the procedure Kelly is about to undergo is not without risk. The greater the number of fetuses, the greater the risk. According to national statistics, when reducing from four to two, or three to two, there is about a 10 percent chance of miscarriage by twenty-four weeks. In other words, for every one hundred women who reduce, ten will lose the entire pregnancy.

There is a terrible randomness in who is forced to choose selective reduction. Two couples with virtually the same case can have the same fertility treatment and one will go home with one or with no baby and the other couple will go home pregnant with four. Lying on the table, Kelly wishes she were someone else. Her first act as a mother is to protect the health of her children, and she is doing just that for two of them. She knows it is right. But she is crushed with guilt, and with the loss of a daughter. The medical staff who do these procedures say every woman cries the entire time. Kelly is no different.

In a reduction, the doctor, guided by ultrasound, injects potassium chloride into the heart of the fetus. The compound interferes with the electric system of the heart and prevents it from beating. The gestational sac will shrink and be partially or totally reabsorbed by birth. In the procedure, the doctor uses two ultrasound monitors. One is used to guide him, the other to show the parents before and after. The parents' monitor is turned off during the procedure, which takes five to fifteen minutes. Then, another ultrasound is done to confirm the ongoing pregnancy. All of this happens as planned in Kelly and Mark's case.

At home, Kelly gets into bed and cries for the next twenty-four hours. Mark tries to comfort her, and he is grieving, too. He tells her to remember the twins she is carrying. He tells her they need their mother. Few things in life are as bittersweet. Kelly and Mark had gotten everything they hoped for. And everything they feared.

Our staff psychologist, Shelly Tarnoff, talks to patients about the many risks of high-tech pregnancies and says that one of the biggest is when a potential brother or sister has to give up his or her life to save another. Sometimes, she tells them, it is only through their spiritual resources that they can make any sense of this. She tells grieving parents that this child they have lost must be remembered and honored for his or her unselfish gift. She advises parents like Kelly and Mark that they must first allow themselves to feel the grief and when they think of the pregnancy, urges them not to deny the reduction but to admit the anger, sadness, remorse, and regret that is a part of it. The next step is to try to get help with those feelings, not from each other, but from other people who support each of them, and to acknowledge what a sad and painful event such a loss represents. The most helpful support comes from those who can nurture each parent and recognize that sadness is part of the normal grieving process. Patients must grieve, Tarnoff says, and also need to forgive themselves. No one can predict when a major multiple pregnancy will occur or what decisions the parents will have to face in light of that. Finally, Tarnoff advises parents to make the lost child real and acknowledge his or her existence, however brief. As hard as it is to say good-bye when they've never said hello, Tarnoff often tells patients to greet their child, and symbolically acknowledge him or her with a letter, put their embryo photo in a baby book, or buy a figurine as a tribute and put it on the mantelpiece.

Acknowledge, celebrate, and honor the life lost. That is where healing begins.

Postscript

At a routine doctor's appointment in November, after Kelly left my care, the ob/gyn expressed some alarm.

"Can't you feel that?"

"Feel what?" Kelly asked.

"That's a contraction you're having."

It was crazy, Kelly thought. She wasn't due until spring, and here it wasn't yet Thanksgiving. The doctor ordered her immediately onto complete bedrest. Kelly stayed on the couch while Mark cleaned the house, shopped, cooked, and then cleaned up their Thanksgiving dinner. By Sunday night, she was upgraded to "partial bedrest," which allowed her to get up three hours a day. She remained on that bedrest for more than a month. It was the year that everyone she knew got a Christmas card. She had to keep herself occupied, and it was the perfect task.

The Friday before New Year's Eve, as Kelly got up to go to the bathroom, she felt a rush of water. Her water broke. It was December 29. The babies were due March 30. Mark got her coat and bag and drove her quickly to the hospital.

There, she was given strong medication to relax her uterus and postpone labor. Forty-eight hours passed. Then, on New Year's Day, Kelly spiked a fever, and her lungs began filling with fluid. The doctors said they had to deliver immediately. Kelly's doctor was out of town. Everyone they knew was out of town.

A neonatologist came into Kelly's room before the scheduled cesarean section to brace the couple for what lay ahead. Infants at twenty-seven weeks gestation are so tiny and fragile that they need to be on ventilators. He said there was potential for many problems, but he wanted Kelly and Mark to think positively and to save their energy for the coming days. He believed the twins had a good chance of surviving.

Shortly after 3 P.M., Kelly underwent a cesarean section. The baby whose bag had ruptured was a tiny baby boy, a mere two pounds, three ounces, but he was doing well. The larger boy, at two pounds, seven ounces, needed far more care. He had been happily floating in fluid, and so was unprepared for his abrupt change in environment. Kelly caught a glimpse of her babies before they were taken to the neonatal intensive care unit. It was the first good look Kelly had of her smallest son. He lay on his back, his tiny legs splayed open like a frog, intravenous tubes running everywhere, patches covering his eyes. Her little James. She realized in that instant that what other parents say is true. "You can't even fathom that kind of love until you have your own children. You can love each other, you can love your family and your parents, but it's a whole different game when it's your child." He was so helpless and vulnerable that Kelly could only weep. Why couldn't she have carried him longer, what could she have done differently? She hadn't even been a mother one day, and she'd blown it.

When the bigger baby, Henry, was ten days old, he blew a hole in his right lung because of the prematurity and had to have a tube inserted. His lung was reinflated and the fluid drained off.

Mark was a rock, working full-time and driving Kelly to the hospital daily, carrying an ice cooler of breast milk. Each teaspoon of milk the babies swallowed was a major victory. They waited for all the complications they'd been warned to expect: bleeding on the brain or a detached retina. Finally they closed the preemie baby book and said if they needed to know about this they'd learn it, but right now, it was scaring them to death. They didn't need to know. Through the days ahead, the boys grew stronger and bigger. On March 26, 1994, Kelly's girlfriends threw her a baby shower, and the nurses insisted she take a day away from the hospital to attend.

"You'll never get another day off," they said.

They were right. On March 27, three days before their due date, the boys came home at more than five pounds apiece. Kelly and Mark went from getting eight hours of sleep a night to getting ninety minutes. The next night they got an hour. But they hung on, and so did the boys.

The boys are named after their grandfathers, who met on the burned-out streets of Berlin all those years ago, and whose reunion brought Kelly and Mark together. The boys are four now, the tallest kids in pre-school. Also the busiest, their mother has not sat down in four years.

While the boys walked, sat up, and crawled well after their peers, they've since caught up. Baskets of books fill their play area. Their parents know they are at increased risk of learning disabilities, but they feel they've been incredibly lucky so far.

Raising twins is a challenge. When one gets a cold, both get a cold; they sleep on different schedules, make every outing an undertaking, and trade personalities and food preferences as frequently as socks. Driving home one day last summer, I passed Kelly and Mark pushing their double stroller and invited them home to meet my wife, Miriam. The four of us stood in the living room watching these busy little boys, the perfect images of their parents.

In this neighborhood, Kelly is no longer the Shot Lady. She is Henry and James's mom, and it is hard to imagine her without the boys, as she throws balls, passes out baseball caps, and calls races. Next summer, she might even go camping.

11 In the Desert

*S*alt hurt. Chips, pretzels, that sort of thing, burned the canker on the side of Susan's mouth. A canker, really a raw spot, a bloodred blotch right on the gum. Anyway, she went in to have it examined at the clinic at the Midwestern college where she was a counselor.

The dentist took a look—Susan'll never forget it—and he stepped back, away from her chair, eyes widening. He walked down the hall to ask the oral surgeon to have a look. And the oral surgeon called the dermatologist so the three of them were just standing there staring at her canker. Now what was going on?

The condition was leprosy-like, of biblical proportions. Susan's immune system was attacking her own cells, launching an all-out assault of the mucous membranes so that the tissue of her nose and throat and vagina began to break down. Blisters spread across her back, becoming open, oozing sores. They wouldn't heal. She'd get into bed with her husband Harry's shirt on—a white long-sleeved cotton men's shirt—and by morning, she'd have to get in the shower to remove it because her skin would peel right off.

The inside of her mouth continued to disintegrate. Susan could barely eat. Her clients would often stop midsentence and say, "Your mouth is bleeding." She never knew where on her body the sores might open up next. When the oozing and sticking got bad enough, she'd wind Saran wrap around and around her torso, dress, and go on to work. She was like a house with no walls.

The diagnosis was pemphigus, a rare and puzzling autoimmune disease in which antibodies separate the outer layer of skin from the inner layers. The cleft formed by the separation fills with fluid, and blisters develop. Before cortisone drugs such as prednisone were discovered to treat this condition, the disease was almost always fatal. Sufferers died of massive infection, like burn victims.

Susan wasn't going to die, but she was going to have to learn to live with her condition. She was grateful because, in spite of the agony that came with the disease, her search for a cure for the pemphigus took her to the Mayo Clinic in Rochester, Minnesota. And those trips, in turn, took her to our center in San Francisco. Because to Susan, having pemphigus was nothing compared to not having a baby. The disease led her to the people who would connect the pemphigus to her and Harry's infertility, the source of her greatest pain.

When it became obvious that Susan and Harry couldn't get pregnant, the high school sweethearts went to the doctor, who found nothing obvious. They tried clomiphene, four intrauterine inseminations, and two in vitro fertilization cycles at the closest clinic. It was 1989. Susan assumed the fertility treatment would work as advertised. It didn't. Month after month the couple tried to have a baby. Month after month her period would start like some sort of small death.

Susan's pemphigus diagnosis was made amid the couple's attempts to conceive. She took the steroid prednisone to control her pemphigus, and it changed her appearance, thinning her arms and legs and bloating her face. The angry eruptions of disease would quiet as suddenly as they came on, but the condition never went away. Susan always had a sore somewhere on her body. She had gone to the Mayo Clinic for the first time to be examined for the pemphigus, when it occurred to her that she and Harry could pursue fertility treatment there. She underwent another two more in vitro attempts, with no success. In the couple's last cycle, the protocol did not include Lupron to prevent inopportune ovulation. When it came time to retrieve Susan's eggs, the doctor discovered she'd already ovulated. All the eggs but one were lost. The lone fertilized egg transferred did not implant. It took fifteen hours to drive to their home from the Mayo Clinic, and Susan and Harry wept much of the way.

As they did after each failed attempt, the couple would retreat to their home and careers, regroup their energy and finances, and then renew their search for a fertility treatment. When Susan first raised the idea of using a surrogate to try to have a child, Harry was open to the discussion. When she got a referral from her Mayo Clinic doctor to a fertility center that offered such options as surrogacy and egg donation, he said fine. Even though it was our center nearly twenty-one hundred miles away in San Francisco and the treatment was not covered by health insurance, he said, "Let's go for it."

A friend once likened the couple's marriage to a Fourth of July parade: Susan was always in the street marching and performing. Harry was always on the sidelines cheering her on.

Susan and Harry had broached the subject of surrogacy with their younger sisters and women friends, who had, over the years, offered their help. All declined, mostly because of the drug protocol. That's when Harry's sister, Jane, thirty-eight, volunteered. She was fourteen months older than Harry, a single mother who was raising two daughters in a small town a few hundred miles north of their city. Jane's daughters supported the plan, as did her doctor, although he warned that in her hometown of two thousand, people would talk. Jane figured she could handle it.

In gestational surrogacy, Jane would carry an embryo created from Susan's eggs and Harry's sperm. Jane would be the biological but not the genetic mother. The three of them teasingly referred to Jane as "the suitcase" that would deliver "the package." Jane underwent a series of psychological and physical tests at our center where she must have been asked 101 times, Can you let this child go?

"I'm going to give you an analogy," Jane told the psychologist. "It's like I'm baby-sitting. After nine months, I don't have to baby-sit anymore. I'm housing this baby until it is old enough to grow on its own." The psychologist, and our medical staff, gave Jane, Susan, and Harry the green light.

At home, before the egg retrieval and transfer took place, Jane talked openly about their plans. In response, friends filled her business office with figures of African fertility goddesses and stones from a nearby beach that is famous for the number of teenage couples who conceived babies there. Others openly disapproved. One woman spat on Jane in the post office and said she was interfering with God's work. Jane, who believed she was doing the right thing, was not shaken as much as flabbergasted by the reaction. Rumors circulated that she was doing classic surrogacy; in other words, that she would be inseminated with Harry's sperm and thus be both the surrogate and genetic mother. "With my brother!" Jane said. "Arrgh."

Susan, Harry, and Jane flew to San Francisco in February 1994. The bad news was that very few follicles had grown, despite a strong fertility drug protocol. Susan's eggs were mixed with Harry's sperm. The four embryos that resulted were fragmented, their cells irregular in size and shape. The doctor transferred all of them into Jane.

Jane returned home knowing she was pregnant. She looked at the changes in her body, and she knew she was. She remembered the feeling from carrying her girls, her bustline was fuller and more tender; she was weepy. It was pregnancy with all its heavenly hormones. That the symptoms were due to the hormones she was injecting to support the pregnancy and not due to a growing baby never occurred to her. But that is what was going on. The pregnancy test was negative. There was no baby. When Jane learned the news, it took a long time to pick up the telephone to call Susan.

That was when Susan and Harry began considering one of the only treatment options still untried: egg donation.

Obtaining eggs from a young, fertile woman to fertilize in the laboratory and transfer into the uterus of an infertile woman was first reported in 1983 by an Australian team led by embryologist Alan Trounson and physician Carl Wood. In November 1983, a baby boy was born to a woman with premature ovarian failure, who had become pregnant with eggs from an anonymous donor. Within two years doctors were reporting using egg donation to help women in their forties and with unexplained infertility to conceive.

To give up one's genetic connection to a child is a huge step. From the time that she and Harry started fertility treatment, Susan felt as though she'd been leaving parts of herself behind. She left behind her privacy, her independence, her control of her own body, when she began treatment all those years ago. When Jane agreed to help them, Susan left behind her dream of carrying a child. Now she faced the prospect of having to give up using her eggs, her unique genetic contribution to her child. Susan thought about the twenty-three chromosomes carried in each egg, the strands of DNA that carry the slightest, dearest frailties, the tendency toward big feet, dimples, those clear blue eyes. She asked herself, What is a mother anyway? Do genes make the mother? Can you be a mother without a child? Susan knew she wanted children. The question that kept her awake at night was how much of herself did she have to leave behind?

The more Susan thought about it, the more she realized that infertility is like driving through the desert and having your car break down. You tinker with the car, and when that doesn't work, you start walking. As you head toward town, you take your purse and your bags with you because you'll want them when you arrive. But as you walk in the killing heat, you start leaving things behind, just to survive. You realize that what you thought was valuable once and what you need to get where you are going are two different things. Susan began to see that she would leave almost every vestige of traditional childbearing behind in order to be a parent.

Susan and Harry contacted the agency that recruits egg donors and surrogates for our patients who require those services. The agency has about 130 donors ages twenty-one to thirty-three, known only by a first name, who are willing to undergo ovarian stimulation and donate their eggs. The donor is reimbursed about $3,000 for her time and effort, as well as for any travel or medications.

At home in the Midwest, most people don't have any idea what Susan and Harry are going through.

"Isn't it about time you two started thinking about having a baby?" a friend asked Harry. When Harry confided they had been trying, it became a topic of some discussion among the guys at the mill. One coworker offered: "You and Susan just need to relax." Another suggested a vacation, a warm-weather trip. "Just get a bottle of good wine, and it will happen." "I'll come over and do it for you," said one father of four. "Because it's obvious I know how." One day a neighbor introduced Susan at a party. "This is Susan; she doesn't have any kids, but we let her stay in the neighborhood anyway." Susan just laughed and excused herself. She found Harry, and he immediately understood how upset she was. He took her hand, and they walked home.

The packages from the agency arrive shortly after this, by post. Five folders, profiles of five women. Susan and Harry read the profiles front to back, silently, at the kitchen table, and then carry them into the bedroom, climb into bed, and read them again. When it comes time for the decision, they both point to their first choice. It is what a social worker would call a "kismet" moment, because they both choose the same one. The donor they like is twenty-three, has blond hair, German and Irish blood, fair skin, blue eyes, medium height, and an education. "Celeste" lives nearly two thousand miles away, a fact they both find immensely appealing. The fertility clinic has attached a cautionary note to her profile, though. She has a long-term contraceptive implant in her upper arm, and it may be a while before it can be removed and she's available. For the woman who will donate her eggs so that they can have a child, they're willing to wait.

In their previous trips to the center, Susan and Harry had worked with various doctors. I meet them for the first time when they come to San Francisco to prepare for an upcoming transfer.

As we talk, I remember how similar accents and sentiments greeted me when I first arrived in North America. When I first immigrated to Canada, I moved to Saskatchewan, a province almost as big as Texas, with no natural boundaries or shortages of water or wheat. You could not say the same of doctors. Anytime overworked doctors took a well-earned holiday, a substitute was recruited to step in. Which is how a South African doctor working in England came to step onto the tarmac at Saskatoon International Airport on February 22, 1981.

I took a breath, and I nearly died. It was sixty degrees below zero, and the dry air hit my lungs like a fist. Inside the small airport terminal, with steamed-up windows and ice-slicked floors, I stood waiting for the daughter of my future partner to collect me. I was nodding and smiling as other bundled-up Canadians pulled off mittens and stomped snowy feet, collected relatives and luggage and departed. Finally there was almost no one left except a young woman. She approached.

"Dr. Zouves?"

"Yes."

She apologized. She explained that she had been told to look for a physician from Africa. She had assumed he would be black.

Like many of my South African medical school classmates, I'd wanted to do a "locum tenens" in Canada, to replace a doctor on holiday. It was a job that offered practical experience and opened the door to eventual immigration to Canada or even to the United States. I had been living in England, where I'd completed fellowships in obstetrics and gynecology and general surgery, a total of nine years of training. I'd already begun doing paperwork to emigrate to the United States when I got a call from a Dr. Alan Gale of northern Saskatchewan. He wanted me to join nine physicians who served the small community of Nipawin and covered the Canadian and Cree settlements surrounding it. Their territory included Cumberland House, the oldest permanent settlement in Saskatchewan built by the Hudson's Bay Company in 1774.

"We have five thousand people in town, fourteen thousand in the area, and we need a physician to come and work with us," Gale said.

Nipawin is nearly three hours north of Saskatoon, on the banks of the North Saskatchewan River. Looking at a map of Canada, Nipawin would be close to the middle of nowhere, in a province that contained, that year, fewer than three people per square mile.

"We'll guarantee you'll receive $96,000 Canadian dollars," he said.

It sounded, to my ears, like a fairy tale. I was earning the equivalent of a quarter of that in England.

Driving north along the Saskatchewan River that February, the prairie was white on white, layered with white. The blacktop was gray. Welcoming visitors entering town was a signpost "The Churches of Nipawin." The churches numbering seventeen, included Ukrainian Greek Orthodox and Ukrainian Catholic. Also eight fraternal lodges and twelve service clubs. The Bible Belt, I thought.

I was the new surgeon and quickly went to work operating four or five days a week, repairing hernias, performing hemorrhoidectomies, removing lumps and bumps, and clearing obstructed colons. I delivered babies and, as part of my rounds, visited the nursing home where the area's oldest residents lived.

In England, I performed surgeries at volumes unheard of in North America, except maybe at shoot-'em-dead hospitals like Cook County.

And already it had begun to change me. Every patient there felt like a case in which I had to "cut it out or cut it off." Patients became "the breast," "the colon," "the gallbladder," and no matter what I did, they often died.

But in Nipawin, my patients were my neighbors. Almost everyone whom I treated in the office, I eventually came to see outside as real people. I saw the wife, the husband, the kids, the grandparents. I performed vasectomies on men who'd lost their jobs in the 20 percent unemployment that crippled most of Canada that year, and I patched up their children who had caught a baseball in the mouth. I remember my elderly neighbor inviting me into her cellar to select preserves she'd put up that year. Her kind, weathered face urging me to take more. Breast cancer.

I learned that she and other patients who faced the worst prognoses had the right to know. Doctors who kept bad news from a patient "for the patient's sake" were patronizing because they had not dealt with the issue themselves. Though I meant to stay in Nipiwan six months, I stayed two years. I left to complete my specialty training in obstetrics and gynecology at the University of British Columbia. But the years in Saskatchewan are among my fondest. I met couples like Harry and Susan during my time there. How far the two of them had come to be sitting across from me now in San Francisco. I knew they must have put everything they had, emotionally and financially, into trying to have a baby.

By now, Susan and Harry have abandoned the surrogacy approach after the cycle with Jane failed. Once it became clear that Susan may have an egg problem and not an implantation problem, they decided to use an egg donor and transfer the resulting embryos into Susan's body. I am using an ultrasound to monitor the thickness of Susan's uterine lining in order to schedule when that transfer will take place.

Their donor's—"Celeste's"—stimulation and egg retrieval are excellent. Three days after the retrieval, the laboratory reports there are twelve embryos. I am meeting with Harry and Susan that morning to make some good decisions about how many embryos to transfer back.

After so many failures, Susan and Harry want to be aggressive. She is on prednisone and seems healthy, her pemphigus is quiet now. The

steroid she is taking to control it seems to be keeping any serious out-
break at bay.

We decide, on the basis of their five failed cycles and willingness to
reduce, to transfer seven embryos and freeze the remaining five for possible future use. Susan and Harry leave the transfer and spend the next
few days resting. They take the two-legged flight east, where they land
and drive home in record cold temperatures.

Ten days later, on Christmas Eve, the blood tests indicate that Susan
is pregnant. When she gets the call, she cannot believe it. Pregnant. The
word swells and fills their mouths, their conversations. She and Harry
tell everyone. Prospective grandparents, the guys at the mill, her clients.
The tests show that the levels of pregnancy hormone in her blood are so
high, it's probably twins. Their long years of imagining this pale next to
the reality of their actual joy.

Then, at six weeks, their local laboratory calls our center. Blood tests
to track the rise in pregnancy hormones week after week indicate Susan
is no longer pregnant. When I receive the numbers from the two previous weeks, I'm sure there has to be a mistake. I call the lab myself. They
double-check. They tell me there is no mistake.

I call Susan to ask her to go in for a repeat blood test and ultrasound.
Her file sits on my desk in San Francisco all that day, while thousands of
miles away, I know she is having the worst afternoon of her life. I feel
heartsick.

As she goes into the ultrasound examination, she is quizzical and dis-
believing. The technician tells her there is nothing apparent in her
uterus. No embryo sacs. No heartbeat. No baby.

"How can there be nothing?" Susan asks. She goes back to her office
and asked a coworker and her son, "How can there be nothing?" Later
she would remember hardly anything of what happened during the following days; in clinical terms, she disassociated. She detached.

I reach Susan and Harry at home that evening. What could I say? I
tell Susan it is unfair. As I talk, Susan makes a terrible, anguished noise.
Harry takes the phone away from her, we speak a few minutes, and he
hangs up. This is the worst, Harry says. He has a sunny personality,
always the friendliest, most easygoing guy on the block, and this has rat-
tled him. He tells himself he has to be calm and strong for Susan,
because if they both get down, they may never get back up.

When Susan's period starts, it seems unbearably heavy.

"Why didn't it work?" people ask Harry. "What happened?"

"I can't answer that," he says. "The doctor can't answer that. Maybe it was never meant to be."

What happened, I believe, has to do with the pemphigus. The autoimmune disease flared ten days before the final blood test, destroying the pregnancy.

We know that women who have other autoimmune disorders in which the body attacks its own tissue, such as thyroid disease, lupus, and rheumatoid arthritis, have more miscarriages than women without such conditions. Most immunologists agree that there is a link between a woman's immune system and higher rates of miscarriage. But there is much controversy in reproductive medicine over how immunological problems affect fertility and exactly what the role of immunology is.

I was using IVIG for patients with autoimmune diseases such as Susan's pemphigus as early as 1992. I consult with an immunologist in San Francisco to go over my proposed plan to use immunoglobulin for Susan as well as heparin and baby aspirin. After our conversation, I feel I can offer Susan and Harry some hope.

I call Susan and Harry to tell them we have three clear options. First, we can take the five embryos we froze after the last transfer, thaw them, and transfer them into Susan. Second, we could transfer them into Jane, their surrogate. Realistically, we can expect only about three or four of the eggs to survive the thaw, and experience tells me we'd need to transfer more into Susan to have any chance against the pemphigus. So our third, and most aggressive option, is to have the donor undergo a new cycle and then transfer the fresh embryos into both Jane and Susan. It is an all-out effort to see if between these two women we can get a single healthy baby.

I tell them to take their time in deciding if this third option is for them. Susan and Harry need to know they could end up with no babies or, if both transfers are successful, they could wind up with four babies. But they also need to consider the cost of the attempt. Susan and Harry are tapped out. They must consider that they've emptied their savings and cashed in their retirement accounts to pay more than $100,000 in an attempt to have a baby. They've mortgaged their house so that they owe more now than they did when they bought it ten years ago. As the discussion begins, Harry and Susan's extended family begins to split along two lines: those who oppose further treatment, and those who support the impending procedure. Parents and siblings who oppose it worry that the couple is investing far too much. Even Harry's parents, who've always encouraged their attempts, fear the young couple is spending everything and will end up with no money and no children. The rounds of treatment have already changed every relationship Susan and Harry have.

Susan finds herself avoiding her mother, her sister, and those friends who argue against proceeding. She is so emotionally fragile that she needs to protect herself in every way possible.

"Either you are on my side and supporting this mammoth effort, or I can't have you in my life," she says. "There is no place for negativity at all."

Even Harry, whose support to this point has never wavered, feels divided. He tells her this is going to be the last time. He tells her that they can't afford another attempt, and that he is worn down.

When I speak to them ten days later, the couple has decided to go with option three. They want to use the same egg donor and transfer the embryos into both Jane and Susan. The agency staff contact the anonymous donor the couple knows only as "Celeste." She agrees to help.

In March 1995, we begin to synchronize the cycles of the three women, ages twenty-five, thirty-eight, and thirty-nine. Susan will take immunoglobulin treatment, a three-hour intravenous infusion, the week before the transfer and then once a month throughout her pregnancy. She'll also take a baby aspirin a day and twice-daily shots of heparin to prevent clotting in the developing placenta. We will boost her maintenance prednisone from 10 to 25 milligrams a day to control her pemphigus.

Jane decides to take her annual leave from her job in community economic development to stay with Susan and Harry in the weeks leading up to their trip. That way, Harry can give the two women a series of estrogen and progesterone shots to prepare their bodies for the transfer. The three of them keep one another company, and their spirits are high. Then, they fly to see me in San Francisco.

Susan and Harry never meet Celeste, whose role in all of this is vital but anonymous. Once again, Celeste's stimulation and response are superb. After her eggs are combined with Harry's sperm, there are fourteen embryos available for transfer. I tell Susan, Harry, and Jane this, and we decide to split the good seven and transfer them into each. Jane is nervous about the higher number and wonders how she'll really feel if she has to reduce. Susan cannot imagine that this will ever be a possibility.

We progress to the procedures. The women are in transfer rooms next door to each other. Harry is so nervous that Susan doesn't want him in the room with her, and asks him to go run errands instead. The transfers go well. Both women lie quietly for an hour at the center, then spend the next day resting in adjoining hotel rooms with Harry administering TLC. They fly home hopeful but subdued.

Ten days later, one set of blood tests comes back positive. The other is negative. The hormone level that should be doubling goes from 11 to 47. I am very pleased to see these numbers.

Aha, Jane is pregnant, I'm thinking.

No, it's Susan. Jane's blood tests indicate that she is not pregnant. Susan is.

"But I don't feel pregnant, and I don't look pregnant," Susan tells the nurse on the phone. Her levels continue to rise, from 453 to 2,074 at her weekly tests. Susan is afraid to let herself believe it. She and Harry don't tell a soul. They go to a fortieth anniversary party that evening, and all Harry wants is for his wife to go home and lie down. At her home to the north, Jane has learned that her test is negative. But she is too distraught to call Susan and Harry. She has gained twenty-five pounds, feels hormonal mood swings, and just wishes she didn't feel so empty.

All eyes, and hopes, are now on Susan. She leaves for work early once every week to repeat the pregnancy test. Naturally most women who become pregnant don't have another blood test once a pregnancy is confirmed. Susan must go in for a test week after week; it feels like a miniseries playing out with each blood draw.

She watches her sisters-in-law one night at dinner. Laughing and talking. They are so confident with their children. Infertility has made her so she is unsure and insecure about everything. She moves like she's on ice—small moves, humble and respectful. She is no longer like anyone she knows.

Before the six-week ultrasound to confirm that there is an ongoing pregnancy, Susan prepares for the worst. She makes a mental to-do list: cancel her prenatal doctor appointment, stop taking medication, call the dermatologist—all things she needs to get busy with when the ultrasound shows nothing. She wants to scream, "I don't even know what's going on inside my body."

"There we go. There's the baby," says the technician, and Susan turns her head, slowly, and there is a baby, blurry; she sees it beyond her tears.

Weeks later, at an appointment with her obstetrician, Susan closes her eyes as he runs the Doppler over her tummy, searching for the heartbeat. It takes a minute. "There it is," the doctor says. Papapapapapap. Susan just lies there and cries.

Postscript

The birth announcement didn't reach me until after the holidays. Joseph was born December 20, 1995, during a scheduled cesarean section to reduce his exposure to the pemphigus. He weighed eight pounds, twelve ounces. Susan and Harry joke that they needed more than one thousand injections to have him. They assume he will look like an ampule. He looks like the two of them.

Two days before Joseph's birth, the mill laid off the last of six hundred workers to be downsized that winter. Harry's supervisor handed him an envelope containing the termination notice just as he headed out on his two weeks of leave. Harry ripped up the unopened envelope in front of the man's face and walked out.

Harry found he couldn't tell anyone. For fifteen years he'd earned a good, middle-class salary, and now, with a newborn, he had no job.

Finally, when Susan came home from the hospital with the baby, he confessed. She was frightened by his despair. She was afraid he'd kill himself. She went back to work counseling as soon as possible to cover the bills, and he stayed home with the baby for eight months. Susan felt as if, just when they'd finally stepped away from the infertility fight, they'd been hit by another blow, an economic one.

Eventually, Harry got on as a part-time corrections officer at the large, regional maximum security prison in their town. It changed him. Within his first few months, he'd cut down an inmate who tried to hang himself. Another day, he broke up a fight by calling to an inmate by name. As the man turned to Harry, his opponent drove a pencil deep into the man's chest. Harry couldn't sleep that night thinking about it. The job pushed the happy-go-lucky part of Harry so deep inside that his friends missed him. After work, before collecting Joseph at the babysitter, he needed to stop at the house to sit down for a half-hour just to bring his blood pressure down. He is looking for other work.

Susan loves being a mother. She started a new consulting company for mental health clients, and sometimes she takes Joseph with her to a group home when she visits. When one elderly resident said she wanted to go home, the three-year-old boy said, "You can't go home. You have to play with us. Here, I'll read you a story."

That she successfully carried an infant to term continues to surprise her doctor. The pemphigus comes and goes.

Joseph's birth helped his aunt Jane, the intended surrogate, get past the disappointment of not getting pregnant. She had learned much about love watching Harry and Susan. She saw how people can come together in a crisis, how a marriage can work. When an old friend called, she agreed to go out with him. They married the following year and are living contentedly with Jane's two daughters.

The egg donor, Celeste, wrote the agency to find out what the baby was and to ask for a photo. Harry and Susan declined. Although she has no legal rights to the child, they are always afraid of her knock on the door. Maybe I watch too much television, Harry would say, but if it happens on television, it can happen in real life. They plan to tell their son the circumstances of his birth as soon as he is old enough to understand. Most of their family and friends are unaware that they used an egg donor. Susan fears that, if they knew, they would treat her baby differently.

After several months, though, Susan wrote to Celeste. She poured her heart out in the letter, thanking Celeste for the child she helped to bring about. He was, Susan wrote, a priceless gift.

I got a letter in the mail myself recently, with a photo of Joseph wearing what appears to be spaghetti. You could see his bright eyes and flushed little cheeks. I consider him one of the most rewarding results I've ever had. The fact that it was Susan who eventually delivered, and not Jane, remains a mystery to me, though. I thought for sure it would be Jane.

12 Giving

A "floater" is the registered nurse who moves between different floors and jobs in a hospital, the part-time position for flexible, mobile, fast-thinking people, someone like Laura. One day she was floating in the newborn nursery when she witnessed a family celebrating a birth. The parents were so thrilled and expansive that she learned in talking to the happy couple that the child was conceived with eggs donated by another woman. A few months later, another woman delivered twins, also from donated eggs. Laura was intrigued by their delight, their ages—they were older—and by their stories. They had long struggled to become parents.

The image of their joy stuck. Shortly after she witnessed that joy, Laura saw an advertisement in a parenting magazine recruiting egg donors, the compensation was $1,500. She asked her husband what he thought. He said he thought it was a scam. But Laura couldn't believe that. When she had her children, her body had worked exactly the way it should have. Laura and her husband had sex, and, as a result, they had kids. Boom. Boom. Boom. Three children. What if she hadn't gotten pregnant? What would her life have been like? When Laura thought of all that her children brought to her life, it was paralyzing to imagine they might never have existed. She also knew what made them really special was that she raised them, not necessarily that they were her genetic offspring. Her own parents had opened their home as foster parents, and Laura had been raised to believe it took more than a gene pool to make a family. She strongly believed that, for it had been the case in her life.

All of this led Laura to contact the egg donation agency. The more she learned, the more she and her husband both agreed it was an endeavor that she should pursue. Laura cleared the agency's psychological and physical requirements and discussions about how she and her husband felt about the process, as well as their feelings on any future contact with the parents-to-be. She filled out an extensive medical and personal history, including her interests and education. She enclosed photos. She was healthy, under age thirty-five, and had at least one child. The proven fertility that Laura provided with these facts is preferable in many egg donation programs.

Laura's profile went into a binder along with those of dozens of potential egg donors. If chosen, she'd be paid $1,500 for her time and trouble. If anyone thought the money was the motivator, they didn't know much about ovarian stimulation, Laura thought.

When she got the call, Laura met the intended recipients at the agency office, where they had a cordial conversation. Most egg donations are anonymous, but this agency's policy was based on openness; they believed it produced commitment, sensitivity, and a better long-term result for all parties.

Laura began the medication to quiet her own menstrual cycle and then a series of injections to stimulate her ovaries. Her husband, who'd become supportive once he learned more about the agency, gave her the shots. Progress was monitored by vaginal ultrasound and the level of estrogen rising in her blood. When her follicles were mature, she was given an injection of hCG to trigger egg maturation, and she traveled to the fertility clinic for the retrieval of her eggs. Several weeks later, she got a call informing her that her recipient was pregnant.

Laura thought she was prepared for that news, but when it came, she had to go into her bedroom for a moment to think about how she felt. She realized that she was happy for the intended mother, who she imagined must be jumping up and down with joy. But that was as far as she could go. She didn't want to know the sex or when the child would be born. Such information would build in her head until it ate her up. She knew she did the right thing by donating her eggs, but Laura didn't want to know any more.

Several months later the agency contacted her again to donate. Again, she underwent the long march toward the egg retrieval. This time, though, there was no pregnancy. Laura felt good about having tried to help a family, but she also figured she was finished taking part in helping others have children.

Laura went on with her life and nursing career; her kids grew. Eventually, she took a job that put her in closer contact with infertile couples. She met other women who were egg donors. About a third were mothers like herself, wanting to share the parenting experience with someone else. Others were educated women, including a doctoral candidate and medical students, who wanted their genes to be passed on but not necessarily to have children themselves. Some donors had had an abortion earlier in their lives, and this was their way of balancing the subtraction, to give a child back to the world.

Laura also came to understand the pain of infertile couples. The ones needing egg donation seemed the most vulnerable, the most victimized by this life crisis. They saw themselves at the bottom of the fertility ladder. At the top of the ladder were people who needed a little assistance to have a family, say, through intrauterine insemination or Clomid. Further down the imaginary ladder were the couples who required in vitro fertilization and got pregnant with their own eggs on the first or second try. Below them were couples needing numerous attempts. And at the bottom, it seemed, were the women who needed another woman to provide the uterus or the eggs if they were to become parents.

Few people understood how much grief there was on the bottom, Laura thought. Women got there through pain. Some had children who died accidentally and now they were too old to easily have any more. Other women had lost their eggs to chemotherapy, or were born without a normal uterus because their mother took DES. Some were just unlucky. Few people outside fertility medicine understood how much time and effort and money it took just to hang on to the bottom rung of the fertility ladder. They didn't understand the decisions made. Least understanding were the fertile, who weren't even on the ladder. They were on the roof looking down.

"I have seen pain so deep and intense, sometimes I have to go in the other room and feel sad about the unfairness of the situation," Laura told a friend. "These are totally loving, together, stable people who have nothing but love to give to a child, but none seem to come."

When a third call came, Laura almost declined. But in the course of the conversation, Laura was moved by the fact that the woman had been disappointed by other donors and was somewhat desperate. She agreed to help one more time.

That summer, Laura and the intended mother start their cycle at our center. First, the women take low-dose birth control pills to synchronize their cycles. Then, daily injections of Lupron to prevent unplanned ovulation. Finally, Laura begins daily shots of fertility drugs. She is taking menotrophins, a mixture of follicle-stimulating hormone and the luteinizing hormone. After seven days of shots and blood tests, a vaginal ultrasound indicates Laura's follicles are nearly ready. She needs an injection of hCG to trigger the final maturation of her eggs and to time the retrieval. The hCG hormone, produced by the placenta in pregnant women and extracted from their urine by drug companies, is similar enough in structure to mimic the luteinizing hormone—the LH surge.

This is a critical time for the donor. If Laura misses the medication that triggers the surge, the eggs may be irretrievable, stuck to the sides of the follicle. Retrieve them too early and they may be immature and fail to fertilize. Too late, and they can be ovulated into the body cavity and lost. At the center, Nurse Anna Hosford reminds Laura that timing is everything.

"You're taking your hCG injection at *exactly* eight-thirty tonight because your egg retrieval is going to be at *exactly* eight-thirty on Saturday morning," Hosford tells Laura. "We need you to be here at eight, we need you to fast from midnight, and we need you to bring a designated driver because you can't drive after having anesthesia in the procedure."

Laura's husband is a firefighter who works twenty-four hours on, twenty-four hours off. Unfortunately, tonight when she needs the shot, he's working. She telephones her best friend, a neighbor who lived through four childbirths and thirty-six years without ever having given anyone an injection. The friend agrees to help. If she fails, they'll have to get to the fire station to have Laura's husband give her the injection.

The two women meet in Laura's kitchen, where the friend practices plunging an empty syringe into an orange once, twice, five times, ten times. She takes a deep breath. She hates needles. The two friends go into the bedroom where Laura cracks open a glass ampule of white powder and one of water. She dilutes the powder in the water, then draws up the solution and pulls down her shorts.

Her friend gasps. Laura looks as if she's been attacked by a subway turnstile. Greenish bruises and blackish puncture points mark where the fertility drugs have been injected deep into the muscles of her hips for a week. She draws a circle with a pen beside one bruise, the target.

"You absolutely cannot go in halfway," Laura directs her friend. "You have to go all the way in. If you go halfway and try and push it, it will just hurt."

Her friend kneels behind her. Laura bends a knee. Her friend bursts into nervous laughter. "I can't do it. I can't do it."

"Just hold it between your thumb and forefinger and pretend you're throwing a dart." The friend takes a deep breath and plunges the needle one and a half inches into the muscle, drawing back a bit to see if there was blood in the syringe, and then slowly depressing the plunger to a count of ten. When she finishes, her hands are shaking. It's almost dark, and, laughing with relief, the two women friends busy themselves disposing of the medication, wiping down the counter, and straightening up until they turn and wordlessly embrace. Outside the window, their children play. The streetlights are coming on. Deep in Laura's muscle, the hormone enters the bloodstream, masquerading as the LH surge that will cause the follicles to bulge out of the ovary, their walls to thin, and the eggs inside to mature for the egg retrieval.

Twelve hours later, and sixty miles away, in our laboratory the embryologist prepares a "house" for Laura. Or rather, for Laura's eggs. The embryologist lays out petri dishes, small acrylic dishes that fit perfectly in a cupped palm. Each will hold culture fluid, a clear liquid full of amino acids, fats, sugars, and vitamins, held at thirty-seven degrees Celsius, body temperature. They rest in an eight-by-ten-inch stainless steel tray about two inches deep that holds the eggs and, eventually, the resulting embryos.

The culture dishes must be prepared the day before an egg retrieval. They are held in incubators that look like hotel room refrigerators, behind one heavy door and one glass door. The eggs are so fragile and the retrieval happens with such speed there is no time for last-minute preparations. When the crucial moment comes, it's all catch and carry.

Thirty-five-and-a-half hours after her hCG shot, Laura comes into the clinic wearing her "fat pants." Having been through a retrieval before, she knows the weight gain is temporary and the result of the size of the ovaries and the stimulation.

Laura dons a hospital gown, empties her bladder, and lies chatting as a nurse hooks her up to an intravenous saline drip. She will receive Diprivan, an anesthetic administered intravenously, that will make her sleep through the twenty- to thirty-minute procedure yet allow her to walk out on her own about an hour later. She'll also receive antibiotics to combat any possibility of an infection. Monitors will record her blood pressure and heart rate continuously.

The retrieval room looks like a mini operating room, the glass-fronted cupboards crammed with boxes of medical supplies, corners crowded with oxygen tanks and intravenous drip poles, a place one might go for any minor medical procedure. Getting to the egg retrieval is a huge journey for the patient, whether she is donating eggs or having her own eggs retrieved. First she must decide to proceed in the first place, then choose a clinic. Next is pretesting and the doctor picking the right stimulation protocol. Then comes the complex series of shots and monitoring of the follicles leading up to the egg retrieval.

Once they're in the egg retrieval room, many patients suddenly feel overwhelmed and begin to cry. The anesthesiologist, who has seen this often, asks Laura about work, making small talk to draw her away from the scene at hand. She is calmly chatting when I tell her to have a nice rest as the anesthesia eases her to sleep.

The next challenge is mine, to get the eggs from the ovary to the lab and to do that with the least amount of trauma to this patient. My goal is to get, if I can, 100 percent of the follicles to yield an egg, and to see that happen in a way that is a positive experience for the patient.

Every woman is unique. Each may make a different number of follicles when stimulated by fertility drugs. The average woman under forty will make twelve to fourteen. The more eggs a patient produces, the more chances the couple has to get embryos. The more embryos they have, the more choice we have to transfer the best of a large pool. The best of the pool has the best chance of growing into a single healthy baby.

Laura is asleep, her journey is almost over.

Mine is just about to begin.

I am looking for the egg.

The egg is thirty-two years old. It has been inside Laura since she was inside her mother. It was surrounded by 5 million other immature egg cells and then the others around it started dying, first by the dozens, then the millions, so that by Laura's birth there was just a million or two left. By the time Laura was in high school, just 300,000 of her eggs remained. By menopause, there'll be almost none.

Each month, in an exquisitely timed release of hormones from the hypothalamus and pituitary glands, the egg cells inside Laura's ovaries begin to grow. They develop follicles, protective bubblelike sacs, that force their way to the ovary's surface. As the follicles grow, the granulosa cells manufacture estrogen, which, in turn, makes the lining of the uterus thicken in anticipation of an embryo. A single dominant follicle emerges and prepares to release the egg and the unique genetic message it contains. When the level of estrogen reaches a peak, a hormone surge causes the egg to float to the center of the follicle. The walls of the follicle thin, open, and release the egg. Some months Laura feels a sharp stitch in her side as the follicle ruptures and she ovulates a single egg.

This month is different. In assisted reproduction, the goal is to produce as many eggs as possible, retrieve them directly from the ovary and fertilize them in the laboratory in the hope that one will survive the transfer, implant in the uterus, and grow into a healthy baby. Fertility drugs replace and exaggerate the normal ebb and flow of Laura's hormones, prompting anywhere from five to forty immature follicles that would normally just die off unused, to mature.

But the egg doesn't drive. No propeller. No thrashing, lashing tail like the sperm. The egg is passive, it can be released from the follicle during ovulation and drawn up into the fallopian tube by its halo of sticky cells and the fingerlike projections of the tube, the fimbriae, or alternatively, aspirated directly out of the ovary by me.

We used to retrieve the eggs under general anesthesia with the laparoscope, inserting a long, thin telescope through the naval to visualize the ovary and then passing an aspiration needle through the abdominal wall to the follicles. For a time, we went through the bladder to get to the ovaries. The bladder is a forgiving organ. But the pain was substantial.

The procedure that I use now is not as invasive and not as painful. I will retrieve Laura's eggs with the transvaginal ultrasound probe, a cream-colored plastic hand tool curved like the nozzle of a miniature gas pump. I gently insert the probe into the vagina where it produces an ultrasound image that lets me see the ovaries and uterus on a television monitor. Mounted on top of the probe is a long, thin aspiration needle to be directed along a dotted line that appears on the image on the monitor.

The lights are low. Laura is asleep, under anesthetic. The image of her pelvis is on the ultrasound monitor to my left. The lining of the uterus looks like a three-layered coffee bean, nine or more millimeters thick. The follicles look like large black holes. Sixteen follicles on the left ovary. Eleven on right I see. Beautiful. Then the retrieval begins.

With my left hand holding the probe, I pass the needle along the top of the guide, rolling it between my right thumb and forefinger, a motion as small and delicate as feeling grains of sand. I pick a spot to one side of the cervix, passing through the smooth pink ceiling of the vagina to a depth of one centimeter and into the ovary on the other side. I control the gentle suction applied to the needle by a foot pump that hums like a sewing machine. I rotate the needle back and forth, pressing gently, so it drills through the tissue. If I were to punch the needle through, I may rupture the follicle and lose the egg. I pick a spot on the center of the ovary and make radial passes from that entry point, emptying the follicles as they move into the line of the needle. My intent is not to go into the ovary more than once. The nerve supply to the ovary is the same as that to the testicle, and I know how sensitive a testicle can be. It makes me proceed as gently as possible.

I rotate the needle into each follicle, apply suction, and the fluid inside rushes out down a long, narrow tube into a test tube containing a thimbleful of culture fluid warmed to body temperature. In the test tube are little floaters, globs and blobs of mucus barely visible to the naked eye, that may contain an egg. The egg is surrounded by granulosa cells, the cumulus through which the sperm will need to travel to penetrate the egg. The halo of granulosa cells around a mature egg is called the corona radiata, the radiating crown. As each follicle collapses, the fluid that flows into the test tube develops a pink tinge as the follicle walls are drawn tightly against one another and the end of the needle. The next follicle, as if on cue, appears directly in front of the aspiration needle, and the process repeats itself.

On the screen, a hair's breath away from the needle, is the telltale wave motion of the iliac vein, the vein that carries blood from Laura's leg back to her heart, and, under it, the artery that carries blood in the opposite direction. We call that vein the "Avoidicus." I've never hit the vein in fourteen years of retrieving eggs from ovaries, and I pray I never will. But my staff and I are prepared to deal with this emergency and open the abdomen if necessary.

The fact is, I love egg retrievals. First, because it is the procedure that gets us to the egg and thus to the embryos. Second, because each retrieval is a technical challenge. I've been doing at least four hundred egg retrievals a year for twelve years and have found that you need absolute focus to have the best hand-to-eye coordination. I used to enjoy a glass of wine on occasion, but I stopped drinking alcohol years ago because I found even with moderate use I wasn't as focused as I wanted to be the next day.

Now, at this point in the retrieval, I withdraw the needle from the empty ovary. Fluid, looking like white puffs of cotton on the monitor, rushes in. The follicle as an egg factory now becomes a progesterone factory signaling to the estrogen-primed uterine lining to expect an embryo in three to five days.

We're all done. As the nurse and I move Laura's legs from the stirrups, the lights come up and Laura begins stirring. In attending thousands of retrievals, my staff and I smile over the fact that the first words out of every patient's mouth as she wakes up from the retrieval are: "How many eggs did you get?"

Laura opens her eyes.

"How many eggs did you get?"

We'll know in a few minutes, I tell her. Her retrieval was excellent. Twelve feet across the room, through a small window cut in the wall, an embryologist takes the last test tube containing Laura's eggs.

The telephone on the laboratory wall rings. The supervisor in charge, Eva Ulehlova, doesn't glance up. She seldom answers the phone.

"What's important is the egg and the sperm, not phone calls," she says.

At the egg table, another embryologist pours fluid from the test tubes into a petri dish swirling a bit and peering at the liquid through a microscope mounted with a green filter. Embryologist Christin Wong is looking for the eggs, too.

By gently swirling the dish, the embryologist brings into view any eggs stuck to the sides. The cells spread out, so that even to the naked eye, the egg appears. It looks like a fried egg actually, the egg white would be the cumulous cells, and what looks like the yolk would be actual egg. The embryologist cleans off any debris or blood cells and moves the egg into a fluid that will nourish it and, with the presence of 5 percent carbon dioxide, hold it at the proper acidity. She prepares Laura's eggs in less than five minutes. She wants to get the eggs into the incubator as fast as possible.

As the hours that the eggs are outside the body pass, the chromosomes in the unfertilized egg become less stable and drift off the spindle. Ideally we do inseminations within two to six hours.

Stainless steel is synonymous with cold, all hard surfaces and angles, harsh reflection and shattering noise. Except here. The in vitro laboratory is a human warming tray; every surface the eggs come in contact is heated. Countertops, the microscope platform, the incubators—all are held at body temperature. The lights are dimmed to a soft rose. Everyone is so gloved and masked, even down to their shoes, that there is a sense that everyone is on tiptoes.

"We keep it warm and dark because that's what the eggs like in the body," says the embryologist. She's never seen Laura, but she knows her history and what will happen to her eggs. Two weeks before Laura's arrival, we introduced Laura's case to the laboratory staff, clinical and coordinating nurses. We also introduced Bonnie, who will receive Laura's eggs after they are fertilized with Bonnie's husband's sperm.

From this point on, the eggs go under the name of Bonnie, the intended mother. So do the resulting embryos. All eggs are identified by the name of the intended mother who will raise the baby. Bonnie's eggs are assigned a specific color, a specific time slot, a specific incubator, one name, one mother, one baby, as simple and straightforward as an umbilical cord. That is the case regardless of whether the woman uses a surrogate, or whether she uses an egg donor and a surrogate. We always have the paper trail recording the egg donor or sperm donor. But in the laboratory, the mother who intends to raise this child is the one whose name is used, to avoid any confusion. From the very beginning, maintaining the identification of the sperm and egg must be an incredibly sensitive and consistent process that demands each procedure be witnessed and signed off, checked and double-checked. Frank Barnes, our executive lab director, calls the laboratory the altar of IVF.

"This is the part we are supposed to get right," Barnes says. "There is no room for error." A large part of his job is making sure there is no loophole in the process that could lead to a mistake in identifying a couple's eggs or sperm.

The eggs Laura made and donated go into the "house" of Bonnie. The nurse goes to tell Laura exactly how many eggs she donated: twenty-one.

By now, the eggs are resting. Laura will soon be dressed and on her way to a birthday party with her husband and children.

Meanwhile, in the laboratory, a white light begins blinking above the door. An employee clad in scrubs, head, feet, and face covered, pads down the hallway to a small window where there is a plastic cup of sperm. On the side, a name, age, date of birth, and signature are written in purple ink.

The road to in vitro fertilization is paved with the egos of men asked to masturbate on hard chairs behind curtains or in a bathroom stall at work. At our center, they produce sperm samples in the Oval Office, named in the early 1990s as a tribute to the gravity of the work performed therein. The Oval Office, actually a pair of offices, is a pair of small lounges with soft peach chairs, glossy *Playboy* magazines, a twenty-two-inch color television, and erotic videos. At the beginning of every in vitro fertilization cycle, we also collect a backup semen sample here and freeze it in the event of "stage fright" on the part of the father on the day of egg retrieval.

We require a fresh sample of sperm the morning of the egg retrieval. The sperm will be mixed or injected into the egg within the next two to six hours. In three to five days the resulting embryos will be transferred into the woman who will carry the child. The fathers who have to produce sperm samples always wonder if there is enough sperm and if it's moving. A new job, stress, turning forty-one—Can that make a difference? they ask me.

"You get up in age, and the body is not as rambunctious," says one intended dad.

I can tell worried men that an illness that involves a high fever or any chronic debilitating condition can and does affect sperm. Turning forty or even fifty does not. I also think that stress must affect sperm counts. It's not the amount of stress that determines the damage either. It's the way a person under stress deals with it that causes the negative effects.

The sperm that the embryologists use to inseminate the eggs can be fresh or thawed from a frozen sample. Frozen sperm, from a donor or backup sample, is held in a small, clear vial and then thawed in a warm-water bath once the eggs are retrieved.

Viewed through a microscope, raw sperm are a living frenzy, all pointy heads and spastic tails. Counting them used to involve painstaking laboratory work. Now, in seconds, a computer can determine the volume of the sample, the concentration of sperm, the concentration of moving sperm, and whether the movement is normal. The centrifuge separates out the slow movers and nonshakers, the dead and the abnormal, leaving the most motile 75,000 per milliliter.

Nearly four hours after Laura's eggs are retrieved, the embryologist draws a few drops of Bonnie's husband's specially prepared sperm up into a narrow pipette and releases them into the fluid holding the egg. The dish is closed, gassed with carbon dioxide to maintain proper pH, and put to bed. Someone in the laboratory has put on a compact disc, and it's not difficult to imagine that there are thousands of sperm and eggs meeting today to the sounds of a jazz saxophone.

In the body, the sperm's journey through the woman's vagina and cervix activate the acrosomes or enzymes in the sperm's head, enabling it to penetrate the egg. In the laboratory, the sperm are activated by washing, centrifuging, and being in a protein-rich egg yolk buffer. Once activated, the sperm begin dissolving the egg's protective layers, the tiny sac in the sperm's head releases enzymes to dissolve the cumulus cells. Then they lash and thrash their way into the thick membrane around the egg, the zona pellucida, shedding the protein coating on their heads, until one pushes a path into the egg's cytoplasm. Once inside the egg, the sperm head separates and pairs with the nucleus of the egg. It is at this stage that the sperm and egg are united.

The next day, the embryologist checks for fertilization. When the embryologist looks into the microscope, she sees the egg is masked by cumulus cells, a halo of cells that would have been dissolved in the reproductive track but that in the lab, must be peeled away. The embryologist uses a series of glass pipettes to strip off the outer cells, drawing the egg into a narrow pipette to separate it from the surrounding cells.

A fertilized egg will have two pro-nuclei, two craters or divots on the egg's round face, a slightly larger one formed by the sperm and a smaller one formed by the egg. The nuclei will form a single cell that will divide into two cells, then four, then eight. By the third day of being cultured, an ideal embryo will have at least six to eight cells. Embryos cultured to the blastocyst stage continue to grow until day five in the laboratory.

Postscript

Three days after the retrieval, the fertilized eggs will be transferred into Bonnie's uterus. Ten days after that, Bonnie will learn she is pregnant. Laura, who knows that this will be the last time she donates eggs, learns of the pregnancy through the agency. She has now helped two families to become families. It's a wonderful feeling. But her experience as an egg donor has made an impact on her family, as well. She appreciates her children and the miracle of their births even more.

Meanwhile, in the laboratory, images of the egg, sperm, and embryo cells appear on television monitors mounted next to microscopes, magnified hundreds of times. These images make most people who work in fertility medicine a little curious about their own gametes.

People who don't work in an IVF lab probably never think about their eggs or sperm. Staff members who haven't tried to have children yet wonder if they're going to have trouble. Others wonder if their partner has good sperm or bad. It's almost an occupational hazard.

"Once you see it, you never look at it in quite the same way," says one embryologist.

13 *Receiving*

*H*ighway 1 snakes along the California coast as is shown on every sports car commercial ever filmed—a driver's dream of twist and turn, bend and dip. Heading down to Monterey in a rented Ford, Susan and Harry bomb south in the sunshine, talking and drinking Smoothies. The couple has traveled back to California to try to have their second child through in vitro fertilization. Their son, Joseph, was born two years earlier with my help, after many years of trying. Because they need to stay close by our center for a week or ten days at a time for monitoring and then procedures, the stay usually includes side trips. One year they went up in a hot-air balloon in San Jose. The next year they shopped in Sausalito. This time it's Monterey.

They stayed too late. At the Monterey Aquarium, they linger too long in the blue glow of the sunfish, orange cup coral, and anemones. They talked too long over jumbo prawns and baby shrimp at dinner. It was dark when they started north. A light mist began falling, and the fog moved up and inland like a gray fleece blanket. In the darkness and the drizzle, it was a different road heading home. The oncoming headlights were blinding, the guard rail gleamed, and on an abrupt turn, the tires skittered onto the gravel and the rental car's rear end came round; Susan looked down, saw the abyss, and thought, the egg donor profiles are on the dining room table. If I die, my mother will find out.

The tire tread caught, tracked, and the Ford roared around the corner. Both Susan and Harry swore and sat up. Harry peered over the steering wheel, ashen. They crept back up the coast to the hotel in San Rafael. In the room, Harry opened the minicooler they carried fertility drugs in and gave Susan an estrogen shot. Susan took her prednisone medication and went to bed. She lay in the dark thinking about the donor profiles that she had inadvertently left in plain sight. That was the thing about secrets. You want to die with them intact.

Their secret was Celeste. A blond, blue-eyed musician. She was so obvious a choice to be their egg donor that the first time they read her paperwork, they both knew she was the one. She had the same medium bone structure and long legs that Susan had, the same hair color, eyes, and heritage. She was twenty-seven and had donated eggs to them twice before. The first time, Susan miscarried. The second time, Susan got pregnant and delivered a son, Joseph.

Susan didn't tell her family about the egg donation at first because her parents disapproved of the fertility treatment, and she didn't want to give them more ammunition. Then, when she became pregnant, she didn't want them to worry. When her son was born, she didn't want them to treat him differently. Now, after all this time, she doesn't know how she would explain everything. Harry always planned to tell his son about the circumstances surrounding his birth, but he didn't want other people talking about it. The same scene recurred every time Harry thought about it. He could imagine little Joseph in a playground fight and someone yelling that Susan was not his real mom.

When they decided they wanted to have a second child, Susan and Harry knew they wanted a full genetic sibling for their son. It made more sense if either child ever had a medical emergency that required, say, a donated kidney. It was also because they adored their son so much. They contacted the agency to inquire if the staff could find Celeste and ask her again to donate her eggs. The staff had a hard time locating the egg donor; it took three weeks. Then another ten days before Celeste's response came.

Harry and Susan knew if she declined, they would not pursue a second pregnancy. Celeste didn't hesitate.

The two women, who have never met, synchronized their cycles and began preparing their bodies for the retrieval and transfer. On an August morning, Celeste's eggs were retrieved and mixed with Harry's sperm. The fertilized eggs grew in the laboratory for three days. Now all that's left is to transfer them into Susan's uterus. Lying in bed the night before, Susan remembered what Celeste had written in her donor profile that had struck so deeply. Celeste's words, written in her own hand, still had their own kind of power.

"If I was in your place, I would pray that the donor was like me. Being the donor I would pray you are loving, supportive parents like I had, and like I want to be. It's not so much for the love of that special little life, but for the love of life itself. How precious it is."

It was nearly midnight on November 12, 1977, when Patrick Steptoe and Robert Edwards examined an embryo from an egg they'd retrieved and fertilized. Lesley Brown lived in Bristol and had blocked fallopian tubes.

"It was beautiful," Steptoe wrote in *A Matter of Life, the Story of a Medical Breakthrough.* "Eight rounded perfect cells. The cumulus cells had broken away and I was filled with awe at the loveliness of this minuscule dot of potential human life." Minutes later, they entered the operating room and transferred that embryo, which implanted and grew into the world's first in vitro baby, Louise.

Twenty years later, in our San Francisco laboratory, embryologists examine embryos in much the same manner. Grading the embryos helps the families select the ones most likely to survive and grow into a healthy fetus and baby. I'm waiting in my office down the hall for their report on the eggs donated by Celeste and fertilized by Harry's sperm.

An hour before the transfer, the embryologist peers through the microscope. An embryo without a hint of a blemish, with divided cells that are even in shape and size, is deemed grade I or "perfect." Next are embryos that have some cell fragments, tiny dark bits on the cells that cover less than 20 percent of the embryo. Its cells are equal in size and shape. Grade I and grade II embryos both have about the same chance of implanting. The third and poorest-grade embryos have obvious fragments over 20 percent of the surface and cells that are uneven in size and shape. The grade III embryos have only one-third the potential for implantation of a grade I or II. More than half the embryos examined annually are of the poorest grade. Forty percent fall into the middle category and a scant 10 percent are perfect, or grade I. The grades become crucial minutes later when the patient and partner enter the doctor's office to decide, as a team, how many embryos to transfer.

Harry and Susan's file lies open on my desk: the chronicle of seven years of heroic efforts to have a baby—four artificial inseminations, six in vitro fertilization cycles, a miscarriage, and one baby, Joseph. Susan has the devastating autoimmune disease pemphigus and for three years has been among my toughest cases. Their files have outgrown three folders and are now organized into two volumes. Now, the file I am studying also contains the results of the embryologist's analysis. The analysis reveals that we have fifteen embryos. None of them is flawless. Seven are good, or grade II; the rest are unevenly shaped or sized and rate a grade III. The poorest, or grade III, embryos have much less of a chance of implanting. But they don't make a grade III baby. They're just less likely, by two-thirds, of making a successful start of the job than grade I or II embryos.

Of course, none of these factors is a watertight predictor; they are simply markers that help my patients and me make choices. Poorer-quality embryos that result from older eggs usually require that more embryos be transferred in order to have a single success. But transferring more than two embryos also opens the door to a possible high-risk multiple pregnancy. I can transfer more than two or three only if a couple will consider selective reduction.

If a couple cannot agree to selective reduction, I have to be really careful how many we transfer. If we suddenly hit the implantation jackpot and end up with three or four or five that implant, it's a nightmare for all concerned, I tell Susan and Harry. Within weeks of this conversation, it will become clear that new culture fluid in the laboratory will allow us to avoid this risk. It is about to become clear that the new medium will allow the embryos to grow in the laboratory longer and reach the blastocyst stage, the twenty- to one-hundred-cell stage of development. A transfer at that stage is closer to what happens in natural conception. We also will see improved success rates because abnormally developed embryos can be more readily indentified. But when Harry and Susan and I speak, we are just beginning to see those results.

Susan and Harry have decided they could consider selective reduction in the small but unlikely event of a major multiple.

"We'll do whatever we need to do to get to where we're going."

"Okay," I say. "As tough as it is, we know we can do selective reduction. We will factor that in. Last time, when you conceived Joseph, we transferred seven embryos and only one implanted. I would recommend a low of four and a maximum of six embryos, knowing what we do about Susan's health and history."

"Five," says Harry, and Susan agrees.

I carry the physician's orders reflecting this decision into the laboratory to give the embryologists the directions personally, as I always do.

In the lab, the embryologist gently moves five of the best embryos into a single petri dish, while another lab worker looks on. She photographs them through the microscope and then returns the culture dish to the incubator to await my call. The remaining embryos will be cultured for another two days, and those that survive will be frozen and stored.

The transfer is being held in the Calypso Breeze procedure room, where Susan lies under pictures of brightly colored tropical birds. Other transfer rooms have similar restful themes to help patients relax. Most partners join their wives for the transfer room, but Susan is afraid her husband's nervous energy would be too upsetting for her. She holds in her hand the small photographic image of the five embryos. She is a little shocked at how many have small blemishes and begins to worry. Before I enter the room, my assistant has prepared her for the procedure. Susan is asked to lie facedown on a special hydraulic bed. Ninety percent of women have a uterus that is tipped forward toward the bladder, so during a transfer, they lie on their tummy with their head slightly tilted down so that the fundus of the uterus is pointing down. In theory, there is less chance that the embryos can migrate back toward the cervix. The hydraulic bed makes this easier and more comfortable. A woman whose uterus is retroverted, tipped toward the back, has her transfer lying on her back.

In my practice, we make every effort to ensure that the same doctor does the egg retrieval and transfer for continuity of care and maximum efficiency, A familiar face is always comforting. The nurses and doctor follow a strict set of procedures around embryo transfer in order to be as predictable and reliable as we can be. I am acutely aware of how vulnerable a woman is when undergoing these procedures. I don't want to do anything to add to her stress. I also feel that physicians underestimate the number of women who have been sexually abused. The transfer is stressful enough without aggravating a past trauma.

With a medical assistant to my left, I kneel on a sponge pad on the floor at the foot of the table.

Susan is doing very well; she's in perfect position. "I'm going to gently examine you now," I tell Susan as I gently insert the warm speculum. I tell her that she may feel me pressing a little on the bladder as I work to get a clear look at the cervix. She is doing great. I tell her that I'm going to rinse the cervix with a saline solution and remind her that afterward, when she is moved, if she feels moisture it is not her embryos coming out, it's just fluid from the saline rinse.

Next, I rinse the cervix with the same solution that the embryos have been growing in. That's to have a continuity of environment for the embryos as they are passed from the laboratory to the uterus. I thread the catheter through the cervix to double-check the route to the best spot in the uterus to inject the embryos. When all is prepared, the medical assistant asks the lab to load the embryos into the catheter. I continue kneeling to wait for them to arrive from the laboratory down the hall.

Let's visualize, mediate, pray, do whatever it is we do, I tell Susan as everyone in the room closes his or her eyes. We're imagining, hoping, and praying to get one or two of the embryos to implant.

In the lab, an embryologist takes the dish holding the family's embryos and draws them one by one into the catheter, a thin, flexible tube with a pink stop tab on each end. She verifies once again under the microscope that the embryos are in the tube. Then, holding them with both hands at chest level, she and an assistant walk thirty-three steps to the Calypso room, where Susan and I are waiting with my assistant.

The embryologist says that the first time she made that journey with the embryos, she was scared to death. She was thinking, I've got babies in my hands. Now, she is just as careful, but less scared.

"The main thing is that people are trusting you to make sure you handle their babies the right way."

"Five embryos for Susan," she announces as she enters the room.

I bend the introducing catheter based on the angle of Susan's cervix, making sure that the catheter loaded with the precious embryos will pass through. Then I thread the inner tubing to about 8.6 centimeters. Susan will feel a little pressure as the catheter goes the final little distance. The tip now rests 5 millimeters from the top of her uterus.

As I hold the catheter, the embryologist puts her gloved hand between mine, her thumb on a small syringe at the end.

"Transfer the embryos," I say. With a minuscule depression of her thumb, the embryos are injected.

"Transferred," the embryologist says.

The assistant clicks a stopwatch to thirty seconds, and we wait in silence. Assisted reproduction combines the expertise of endocrinology, gynecology, pharmacology, embryology, and the technologies of cryo-preservation and micromanipulation. But it is here, in the mechanical transfer of a few cells into a woman's body, that there is room for a mundane mistake. If the catheter goes into the lining or doesn't go far enough, the embryos can be damaged or lost. The more transfers I do, the more I realize how critical a step the transfer is. The embryo transfer is also a very spiritual moment. It's the moment that the genetic material this couple has given over to our care comes back to them. It's a very empowering time for couples, as well. Those embryos have come home, and our hope for everybody is that they come home to implant.

When the stopwatch buzzes, I gently withdraw the catheter, turning it two complete revolutions to ensure that the embryos won't follow its path out. The two embryologists then return to the lab with the catheter to check under the microscope that it's empty.

Susan had no pain during the transfer. Her eyes are closed. She's thinking that these embryos are not part of her, that they're part of the egg donor and Susan's husband, and that she needs to welcome them in. She thinks of a statue of Jesus and Mary where she prays at the chapel near her work. She believes what happens next will be a decision of God.

"All clear," the lab assistant reports.

All right, the catheter is all clear, all the embryos are in Susan's uterus.

She needs to stay very relaxed as we move her into a more comfortable position. She will rest one hour on her tummy, dozing under a warm blanket.

Postscript

Harry and Susan go back to San Rafael, where she lies perfectly still for two days. She telephones Joseph, her preschooler, who is staying at Grandma's. When she first considered using donated eggs, Susan grieved the loss of a genetic connection to her child. But in carrying her son, delivering him, and raising him, that feeling has passed. In a day, Harry and Susan will fly home, and in ten days, they will know the outcome of this journey. They will know that Susan is pregnant. Until then, they have learned, over the years, to wait.

14 Sisters

*J*ulia had no symptoms.

Of course, later she realized she'd had a bunch; but for weeks she dismissed them, overlooked them: having the urge to urinate, her flat stomach pooching out so that she had to unbutton her pants when she got into her car after work, not enjoying sex.

"You don't seem interested," her husband, Richard, would say, rolling away from her.

"It hurts," she said quietly.

The usually soft flesh of her lower tummy felt unnaturally hard. She called Richard into the bedroom one night to show him. He felt the firmness with alarm. She had a Pap smear five months earlier, but thought maybe she should show the doctor. She went in that week.

"Could you be pregnant?" the gynecologist asked, moving her hands across her stomach.

"No. Not yet."

Julia and her husband had just begun talking about a baby. She was nearly thirty, and after eight years in television and ten years in the relationship, she was ready. At her last checkup she'd asked the doctor self-consciously if everything appeared in working order. She was fine, the doctor assured her. Until now.

"This isn't normal," the doctor said, concern in her voice. "This is something very big. We're going to do an ultrasound today. Can you call Richard?" Julia nodded.

On the ultrasound monitor, there appeared what the doctor termed a "large, nonspecific mass." They would have to operate to remove it and determine whether it was cancer.

Richard and Julia left the doctor's office in stunned silence. Walking into their one-hundred-year-old house, Julia went straight into bed, curling her five-foot-ten-inch frame into the smallest ball possible, she was so scared. How could this happen? How could it have happened so fast? How could a journalist so skilled at observing others miss so many signs within herself?

It was early morning in Massachusetts. Light barely peeking through the blinds as Julia's sister, Ivy, gazed into the eyes of her six-week-old son who was sucking at her breast. She jumped when the phone rang.

"Who died?" she said into the phone.

"I might," said Julia.

Ivy listened to her sister's anguished story.

"I'm not going to let you have cancer, Julia," she said. "Have them cut it out, just get it out. If you lose your uterus, I will have babies for you. Just get the damn thing out."

She hung up and began organizing the details, making lists. She'd send flowers, gardenias. She'd send a Marie Callendar pie. She would do anything she could for Julia. She would, in fact, almost die in childbirth for Julia. But all that came later, all that was obvious then was the instinct to fight for her sister, it was automatic, snap fast, as uncontrolled as the tears that wet her face.

They were the best audience the other ever had. When their parents' perfect 1950s marriage ended in the less-than-perfect 1960s, Julia and Ivy slid into the catch-as-catch-can schedule of a single-parent household. Their mother worked two jobs, teaching school every day until 4 P.M. and then heading downtown for a hotel nightshift. Sometimes she'd fall asleep in the car when she pulled into the driveway at 1 A.M. The girls would come outside and shake her awake.

They learned to cook for themselves and think for themselves and look out for each other. They had a baby brother, and when they fought, their mother would say, "Listen! You're all each other has." They grew up inseparable and quite separate from the community they lived in. They were nonbelievers in a Bible Belt town.

As they grew up, the bond grew stronger. They roomed together in college, vetting each other's boyfriends. Then, one morning Ivy boxed up her cookbooks and spices and announced she was moving to New York City to become an actress. Julia took a long time getting over that.

Years later, after they had married and moved on with their lives and careers, their differences became pronounced. Ivy married an Englishman and became an artist and a mother of two. Julia, a journalist headed onto the Career Central track, married a scientist and stayed in their small Western hometown. They lived twenty-six hundred miles apart.

Still, Ivy looked to her sister as her touchstone, her foundation. When Julia looked at Ivy, what she felt was so pure and intense it could bring on a migraine headache.

After Julia went to the doctor, her husband, Richard, went to the university library. "Cancer, uterine; diseases, uterine; tumors, uterine." He grew calmer by the sentence, a biochemist at home in the language and logic of scientific studies and abstracts. He learned that malignant tumors in the uterus are nasty; they kill women quickly. A malignant tumor that size could kill his wife within the year. Still, given her history and age, the odds seemed on her side.

The surgery Julia underwent the following Friday lasted five hours. An oncologist arrived, a pathologist, and finally the gynecologist, who reported that she had removed the uterus and the lymph nodes because the massive growth appeared to be cancer. Richard was silent as he absorbed the news.

Next to him, Julia's mother, Helen, began to shake. Richard turned away from her and walked straight out of the hospital, through the parking lot, and onto a dusty trail that rose through the scrub to the foothills on up into the mountains. He walked faster and faster until the blood was pounding in his chest and his head, and he doubted seriously he had the strength to get through this.

.   .   .

It was not cancer, they learned three days later. Physicians didn't know why the noncancerous tumor grew so fast or why white blood cells were pooled around it in a full-blown counterattack. A slice of the softball-size growth was shipped to a leiomyoma specialist at Johns Hopkins University, who responded that he didn't know either.

The gynecologist sat on Julia's hospital bed and said she hadn't expected to have to remove her uterus. The ovaries were fine, however, and Julia's hormones would continue to be secreted. Around her, the family sighed in collective relief. The loss of her uterus was regrettable to them, of course, but tolerable compared to losing her. Julia lacked their perspective.

She had imagined her life with children. Not in the day-to-day sense, but in the long-term plan, the life plan, in her forties and fifties around dinner tables and Christmas trees and in vacation photos. Smart, happy kids. Richard was wonderful with children. That her loss was now his loss filled her with grief.

She recovered slowly. Returned to the newsroom, to long hours and important interviews. She returned to her career all without returning to her old self. She stopped calling Ivy, stopped making smart-aleck remarks or laughing at anyone else's. Everyone noticed. The change was not subtle.

Helpless, Julia's mother, Helen, visited her old gynecologist. "Is there such a thing as a uterine transplant?" she asked. The doctor gently said no. Nor could Helen carry a baby for her daughter. "Too old."

Richard tried to bring up adoption, but Julia would not discuss it. As a journalist, she had reported stories on the failures of the state's child protective services and she knew a family who had had a terrible experience. No, she said, they had two choices: surrogacy or no kids. They lacked the money for the one and the stomach for the other. Some choice. One night Julia told him he should leave her for a fertile woman. "That's ridiculous," he said. He loved her.

But later he would say he'd be lying if he said that it hadn't occurred to him. It was so impossible to do with her what seemed laughably easy with almost anyone else.

. . .

In Massachusetts, Ivy reached a decision.

"I'm going to have Julia's baby," she told her husband, Jack.

"Of course you are," he said mildly. Anyone who knew her could grasp the logic. Ivy adored her sister. She was also creative and unconventional and good at having babies. Ivy and Jack had two children, who they estimated were the result of exactly three nights of unprotected sex. Ivy's pregnancies were healthy, her labor and deliveries efficient, managed by midwives. No episiotomies, no epidurals, no sweat. She mothered without a manual. She assumed children would eat arugula and pesto and roast chicken, and, sure enough, her children did.

They planned a trip west and scheduled a family meeting.

"You're probably wondering why I've called you here today," Ivy announced when they all gathered. "We're going to have Julia's baby. I'm going to carry it. Richard and Julia will contribute the egg and sperm." She'd be thirty-five in August, Ivy explained to all of them. She didn't want to be pregnant much past that. She was so matter-of-fact, so clear, so certain, that she left Richard and Julia almost no way to say no. It was also the only way, of course, that the two of them could ever say yes. Short of her insistence, Richard and Julia could never have asked for such a life-altering favor. Asking for anything ran counter to Julia's nature. She was the giver: giving of advice, information, money, herself. She had no experience on the receiving end.

They began talking seriously about the prospect and agreed the surrogacy could not cost Ivy anything financially. They determined they needed between $20,000 and $30,000 to cover the cost of retrieving Julia's eggs, fertilizing them, and transferring them to Ivy. Also, they needed money for travel and medications. By the breakfast's end, those who could afford it least contributed the most. Julia and Ivy's mother mortgaged the house she'd raised the kids in. Their father pitched in. Richard's parents joined the club they dubbed "The Investors." Even their baby brother Sam, who was between jobs and living halfway across the country, managed to send $250.

The sisters researched in vitro fertilization procedures, fertility clinics, and the science of assisted reproduction. They scanned the Society of Assisted Reproductive Technology Registry, visited the library, and scheduled an appointment with me at our center in San Francisco. If they were unclear about anything, they thought it was a few ridiculously small details in the whole elaborate scheme. Ivy didn't realize, for instance, that surrogacy involves shots.

Needles, by their nature, inflict pain. Sharpened steel pressed against the skin, puncturing the paper-thin epidermis, the gel-like dermis, the sub-cutaneous fatty tissue, down to the muscles underneath. Imagine the initial sting, the cramping or soreness of the tissues as the medication enters. The slight withdrawing tug. The inevitable bruise.

In vitro fertilization relies, necessarily, on needles. Blood is drawn to rule out infectious diseases and check for immunity. The medications used to stimulate a woman's ovaries, mature the eggs, build the lining of the uterus, and overcome immunological problems, are also adminis-tered by a needle.

"Can we take the drugs orally?" Ivy asks me in a telephone consulta-tion prior to their trip to San Francisco. "No, I'm sorry," I say, "you can't take the drugs by mouth. Injections allow the drugs to reach the blood-stream and be delivered directly to the target organs. If you swallowed them, they'd compete with whatever food is in the digestive system, then be carried to the liver, metabolized, and an altered hormone would then make its way to the uterus."

"Would the shots hurt less if I was fatter?" she asks.

"I don't know," I say.

Ivy will be the gestational surrogate, a host, not the genetic mother to the child she will carry. Such surrogacy has been an option available to women since 1985. It is legal in California, but laws in other states and countries vary widely.

As the surrogate, Ivy, and her husband, are required to go through physical and psychological tests and to talk to a counselor about what they'll do if there is a major multiple pregnancy, a tubal pregnancy, a birth defect, and how they feel about genetic testing. They also talk about how Ivy will feel giving the baby to Julia and Richard after birth. Ivy is adamant that this will not be a problem. She had her two children; she does not want any more. This is about her sister, Julia, and Julia's baby. Julia and Richard undergo testing and counseling, too. Everyone involved is excited.

Of the one thousand in vitro fertilization cycles we perform a year, about sixty to eighty involve surrogates, and of those about half the surrogates are a friend or relative of the couple. Motherhood is inherently sacrificial, but perhaps that is most obvious when a woman deliberately carries a child for someone else. Pregnancy carries risk for any woman, from minor varicose veins or hemorrhoids to losing a uterus or even her life. Counselors who work with surrogates testify to the existence of altruism that they see in these women, a desire to help that is both inspiring and inexplicable. Some women become surrogates for spiritual or religious reasons, others to somehow make up for an earlier termination or pregnancy loss. In Ivy's case, her choice to become a surrogate is out of sheer habit of looking out for her sister.

Medically, to accomplish gestational surrogacy, I must coordinate and replicate in two women what nature does in one. First, we must synchronize the cycles in both women, using the birth control pill and the drug Lupron in order to suppress their hormonal cycles and bring them, essentially, to the starting line. Once both women's ovaries are "down regulated," we'll begin to stimulate Julia's ovaries using fertility drugs. This presents a bit of a sticky wicket. Both Julia and her mother have a history of blood clots. Julia is thirty-one. When she was eighteen she developed a deep vein thrombosis in her leg because she took the birth control pill. I know that as we stimulate her ovaries, we're going to be pushing Julia's estrogen up very high, and I know estrogen can cause a blood clot. So we have to take steps to guard against that. I prescribe the blood thinners heparin and baby aspirin leading up to the egg retrieval and have her continue on those for the two weeks thereafter. Julia is terrified of taking the birth control pill again to begin the cycle, and I tell her we can begin without it. The point is not to kill her with anxiety, it's to give her a baby. Lupron should suppress her natural cycle enough to prevent any inopportune ovulation.

Ivy is worried, too. Because we switch off her ovaries in gestational surrogacy, the pregnancy must be supported by external estrogen and progesterone for the first eight or nine weeks. After that point, all the hormones needed by the pregnancy will be produced by the placenta. The shots terrify Ivy. Her elementary school immunizations played out like hunt scenes, and she was the rabbit. Not much has changed over the years. She is thirty-five and has never donated blood.

Many people are anxious or squeamish about injections. I tell Ivy, as I tell other patients, that she might consider seeing a counselor to learn some stress management techniques and explore the question of whether they can or should go forward. After we speak, Ivy contacts a hypnotherapist in Massachusetts to help her confront her pathological fear. After repeat sessions, they conclude that she's afraid of receiving the wrong medication in the syringe and of being out of control. So Jack and Ivy attack the injection dilemma the following way:

First, Jack numbs Ivy's thigh or hip with a bag of frozen peas. Then Ivy uses guided imagery to put herself on a favorite street in Greenwich, Connecticut, or Paris, at which point she begins slowly counting: one, two, three. On the count of "three," he gives her the shot. With this method, she is in control. Ivy can stop him at any time.

The first needle Jack will use is the Lupron needle, similar to the insulin needle used by diabetics, pin-thin, scarcely a half-inch long, and, according to the literature, "virtually painless." It takes Jack ninety minutes to give her the first injection. He is sweating, and she is crying, and she keeps saying, "Stop, stop." This, he realizes, will be a very long month.

They make the injections a morning ritual to try to get the ordeal behind them early. Soon, though, Ivy begins to dread going to bed. Over the weeks, Jack believes they're getting quite good at it. But when it comes time to give the deeper, intramuscular injections, such as estrogen and, eventually, progesterone, they need to call in the neighbor who is a nurse. Ivy's fear is so primal, so painful to witness, that after a few minutes, the nurse wordlessly wraps her arms around her and just holds Ivy close.

Julia, on the other hand, has no problem with needles. She injects herself while talking to Ivy on the telephone.

It takes a village to arrange the retrieval and transfer. Julia and Ivy's mother, the prospective grandmother Helen, flies east to care for Ivy's family while Ivy flies to San Francisco to meet Richard and Julia. They share a single hotel room to save money.

"Who is snoring?" Julia asks one night, half-asleep.

"You!" Richard and her sister say.

Evidently, the hormones make Julia snore. She's convinced that the combination of hormones also makes her loopy. The drugs to suppress her natural cycle temporarily put her in a perimenopausal state. She gets headaches. Other women say they feel hot flashes. At work, an editor tells Julia that her spelling, grammar, and punctuation are off. All of those feelings end in a few days, much to the journalist's relief.

Even before her cycle began, Julia was concerned about her ovaries being overstimulated, having heard of ovarian hyperstimulation syndrome.

Part of the "art" of assisted reproduction is determining the strength and variety of fertility drugs a woman should take. It's a decision based on her age; her menstrual history; her hormone levels, on certain days of the cycle, of estrogen and follicle-stimulating hormone; and any history of prior ovarian stimulation attempts. I try to reassure Julia that all patients undergoing assisted reproduction have a certain degree of hyperstimulation, that one really cannot stimulate the ovaries without causing some enlargement and some lower abdominal discomfort caused by the ovaries' enlargement. Different women react differently to the stimulation. Some seem to be more uncomfortable during the stimulation part of the cycle than others.

Some clinics automatically choose a light drug protocol during the first cycle. They assume that it's a trial run. But an in vitro fertility cycle is too costly emotionally and financially and time-wise to make the first cycle merely a warm-up. Frankly, I don't want to stimulate too conservatively and end up with a canceled cycle because too few follicles develop. On the other hand, I don't want to endanger a woman's health. What gives me the ability to be aggressive and at the same time to keep this woman safe is the prolonged coast, which keeps the most severe ovarian hyperstimulation syndrome from developing.

Julia produces forty-four follicles, and it is necessary to coast her for six days until her estrogen drops to a safe level. After the egg retrieval, she says she feels pounds lighter. The news from the laboratory is that she produced twenty-eight eggs, twice the average of women under forty. Three days later these eggs become twenty-two embryos, fifteen of which were grade I, or perfect. Ivy starts calling her Chicken Woman, "baaaaak-bak-bak."

Throughout the week, the surrogate, Ivy, is firing off one-liners like an automatic weapon. Humor is her natural and best defense. Daily trips to the center for injections and monitoring all feel very clinical and intense to her. She is anxious about the transfer. When Ivy comes in for the procedure three days later, she makes it obvious she feels like a laboratory rat in an experiment. It's not a subtle hint. She's wearing a gray and pink rubber rat mask.

She takes a seat across my desk with Julia and Richard. I begin the discussion with the embryologists' report as we determine how many embryos should be transferred. An average number to transfer when the egg provider is under thirty-five is three or four. Out of the twenty-two embryos available, we decide together to transfer four perfect six-celled embryos. This entire discussion takes place between all those involved without my acknowledging Ivy's rat mask.

Before we leave my office for the procedure room, I offer patients a Valium to help them to relax during the transfer and sleep during the required hour of rest afterward. Three-quarters of my patients take me up on it, and nearly 100 percent of the husbands say, "I'll have one, too." I always have to say, "No Valium for the husband, he's driving."

Julia has decided to join her sister in the transfer, and a nurse helps Ivy get ready for the procedure. Ivy is placed in position on the hydraulic bed and covered with a sheet. When I come into the transfer room, there is a little giggling, and, as the nurse pulls back the sheet, there is a smiling "Kilroy was here" face staring back at me. Ivy has had her sister draw the large smiley face on her right rear cheek. It's a joke, a sight gag, a way for two very funny women to tough their way through this high-wire act. But I chose not to respond. That reaction may seem cold, but the stress of an in vitro cycle elicits different reactions from different people. This was Ivy and Julia's way of coping, but I am already trying to visualize the catheter's path through the cervix with its precious cargo.

I do the embryo transfer exactly the same way every time. Doing the transfer in a very standardized fashion ensures that there is no ambiguity about commands or the process, and no chance of misunderstanding between myself and my staff. It's also the most respectful way I can think of to treat a patient. The nurses, who are trained in how to approach or move a woman, prepare patients expressly so that I am not doing anything that might be invasive or upsetting. This is an intense procedure—physically, emotionally, and spiritually. The staff must be respectful, predictable, and protective of a woman's dignity at all times.

That's why Ivy can't get me to laugh in the transfer, regardless of her mood or how funny she is. It's a bit like laughing in church. You may feel relief at the time, but you would inevitably question its appropriateness later. But she can't help laughing herself. And I understand this stress-releasing impulse.

When the catheter is in place, I say, "Transfer the embryos."

"Embryos transferred," the embryologist responds as she injects the contents of the catheter.

This exchange sends Ivy over the edge. The exposure she is feeling, the whole surreal sense of the event, and now this formal pronouncement that sounds to her like a *Star Trek* command, are overwhelming. She starts to giggle and can't stop.

Later she tells me she's afraid her giggling shook the embryos loose. I tell her that's probably not possible. The events after each transfer are like the last few minutes of a football game, analyzed by everyone. Every sneeze, every cough, every angry word with a spouse is analyzed to try to attach a cause and effect. It's human nature to understand or account for the unknown.

But I explain that once the speculum is removed after a transfer, the walls of the vagina come together, and, as the floor of the pelvis closes, the muscles at the base of the pelvis contract so the pressure around the uterus is equal. Whether a woman laughs or coughs or sneezes, the net vector is zero. It's like two hands banging on a basketball from opposite sides; they cancel each other out.

Back in the hotel room Ivy takes it easy. She's the gourmet cook in the family, but she sends out for fried chicken that night. It's a meal she's loved from childhood. Comfort food.

At the airport as they depart San Francisco, the two sisters embrace. From the shots to the egg retrieval to the difficult decisions before the transfer, they have done everything within their control to make a pregnancy possible. Now it's out of their control. Ivy flies to Massachusetts with four embryos suspended in her uterus. She tells her sister, "I have no doubt this is going to work."

It does work. A pregnancy test ten days later reveals Ivy is pregnant, and she is immediately protective of the child she is carrying. She eats fresh fruit and drinks milk, skips coffee and diet Coke. On a trip to a southern beach, she doesn't even let the water touch her above the thighs. She is thrilled and hopeful.

.   .   .

One evening Jack and Ivy go to visit friends.

"I think you're playing God for your sister," says the friend. "It's obvious she's not meant to have children."

Ivy looks at the woman's five children and realizes some people will never understand.

Four weeks after the transfer, Ivy begins to bleed and throw up. She throws up violently and bleeds enough to fear she has miscarried. When she calls San Francisco, I tell her not to assume she has lost the pregnancy. She must keep taking her progesterone injections. It's very likely that she is still pregnant.

I get the call from Massachusetts the following afternoon. Great news: Ivy is pregnant with twins.

It was bitter that winter in Boston. Snow fell two, three, four feet deep. Ivy couldn't leave the house for days; she couldn't get the car out of the driveway. Both her preschoolers were sick and whiny, with runny noses and deep coughs. No one slept through the night. At sixteen weeks, Ivy caught the terrible cold herself, and at the next ultrasound, she discovers one of the fetuses has died.

She said that telling Julia was the hardest call she ever made. Her sister sounded like she was on the other side of the planet. Ivy was overwhelmed with guilt and grief and the need to somehow separate her mind from her pregnant body. She had thought she would feel differently about this baby than she did her own. She didn't expect or want to feel the amazing interplay of her earlier pregnancies, the constant internal conversation that a woman has with an unborn child. But this pregnancy felt exactly like her earlier ones.

Each morning she stuffed a used syringe from a hormone injection into a plastic two-liter Coke bottle, an act she'd repeat a total of 107 times. She forced herself to call Julia and Richard with cheery reports on the progress of "your baby" after her prenatal exams.

As the winter dragged on, she felt ungainly and depressed. Ivy wanted to talk; she needed to talk about this swirl of emotions, about this piece of delicate crystal she felt as if she was carrying around inside.

But Jack was either traveling for work, or the boys were underfoot, and anytime she tried to talk to her sister, Julia was flat. Ivy didn't know that Julia was so frightened by the problems early in the pregnancy and so afraid of being wounded once again in this process, that she withdrew, pulling her hope and emotions inside. All Ivy knew is that after talking to her sister, she felt even more alone. Ivy pictured herself as a whale on a beach, stranded.

She found herself talking to strangers. If someone in a grocery store was lucky or unlucky enough to ask about her emerging belly, out came the whole saga; she'd rattle it off in some sort of manic confession. "Wow!" they said. She talked to so many people while shopping at an outlet mall in Maine that, months later, all the clerks were dying to know how the story turned out.

Ivy gained fifty-five pounds and a bright red rash erupted on her face like a Mardi Gras mask. She called Julia to kvetch, to connect with someone who loved her and this baby, who cared what they might be going through. Julia's responses were monotonic, her voice as hard as Western granite. A few days later, Julia was working on deadline when the phone rang.

"Julia, that last check was $1.23 short."

"What?" Julia said, turning her back to her coworkers. "Ivy, what is this about?"

"The check you sent, it was $1.23 short."

Julia felt herself go cold.

"Why are you calling me? This phone call is costing you more than $1.23."

Julia grew colder as Ivy emoted and indulged her feelings, feeding them, exposing them, sharing them, doing all the things Julia would love to do but couldn't. When Ivy told her that she would have this baby with a midwife, it didn't matter that Julia would have preferred she go with a obstetrician, Julia said, "No problem."

When Ivy refused to do amniocentesis, saying there was too great a risk of miscarriage, Julia, who would have preferred to know if there was anything wrong with the baby, said, "No problem."

Julia was trying to be the good soldier and cheerleader. She and Richard paid for Ivy's groceries, for the hypnotherapy sessions, and for a meal service to deliver "depression dinners" to lift Ivy's spirits. Julia found a gynecologist's speculum, spray-painted it gold, and sent it off to Ivy: "The Golden Speculum Award" for "Uterine Service Above and Beyond the Call of Duty." She sent her sister weekly presents of jewelry or fragrance and paid a housekeeper to clean Ivy's house every Wednesday—a luxury she and Richard could never afford.

"They are taking blood out of my arm every week," Ivy said in her ear.

Julia felt a headache so intense she couldn't move. She told Ivy to call Richard about the checks in the future. Then she hung up. "We were not very good friends," she would say about that period later.

Postscript

The baby was due June 17. The whole family flew to Boston for it, and nine days later they were still watching Ivy like an egg timer. Ivy wanted everyone to shut up and go away.

"I've had it," Ivy said after the umpteenth inquiry. "I don't want to see you people."

When she finally did go into the hospital that night, her labor was longer and harder than anyone could have expected. She outlasted Richard, Julia, and Jack as they coached her. Despite tremendous back labor, she delivered drug-free. Her husband said she pushed that boy out by sheer will.

That boy. More than eight pounds perfect. Richard and Julia ripped their shirts off and pressed their son to their chests. Through the haze of tears and blood and relief, it registered dimly in Julia's mind that a crowd of people was gathering around Ivy.

"There's a lot of bleeding," the midwife said. "There's an awful lot of bleeding." Jack watched dumbfounded as the birthing room of casually dressed staff suddenly became a sea of people in surgical masks and scrubs.

"She's losing too much blood; we're going into the operating room."

Ivy's placenta would not detach, and her blood pressure was plummeting. Ivy had never been in an operating room before. The midwife said that they first were going to try to remove the placenta manually and a doctor would operate if necessary in order to stop the bleeding.

Ivy kept trying to visualize her sons and husband, but the blood loss was too great, and she felt herself losing consciousness; at one point she felt herself losing everything and just slipping away.

The midwife was repeating, "Hang on, hang on, come on, come on."

Jack, who thought in newspaper headlines, saw tomorrow's paper: "Woman Dies Delivering Baby for Sister."

Ivy, who believed she was dying, saw nothing at all. She had this idea that when you die, there was something there, heaven, a big condo, a place where you recognized people, where it was crowded. Wherever she went was nothing like that. There was nothing and nobody. It has been a terrible thing to live with ever since. Ivy recovered. She lost two liters of blood and needed three blood transfusions, but eventually her strength returned.

Julia recovered, too. Since she lost her uterus and embarked on the in vitro journey, she knew one thing: If she allowed herself to feel any hope, the hope always coincided with extreme pain. It was the two-headed dragon inside of her: hope and pain. Anytime she fed one, the other one would grow as well. As long as she kept herself flat, and felt absolutely nothing, she could starve both dragons into submission.

Julia's dragons went away the evening after her son, Ben, was born. First she saw that Ivy was going to be all right. And finally, when Julia was alone with her baby, all alone for the first time, she cradled Ben. She held his tiny and smooth body, so small and perfectly male. Then he peed all over her. She laughed so loudly the nurse came.

Richard and Julia adopted Ben in two states. Ivy and Jack were identified as the birth parents. So first, the family got a voluntary denial of paternity from Jack, in order to list Richard's name on the birth certificate in Massachusetts. That allowed Julia to apply for a second party, or stepparent, adoption at home. Richard and Ivy told their hometown judge everything about the surrogacy, and he approved the adoption straightaway. They took their son to a freshly painted nursery in their one-hundred-year-old house.

Ivy and Jack went home to raise their own two boys. Ivy began painting again. The sisters talked on the phone, but the conversations seemed strained and were almost always about the surrogacy. Then one day, more than a year later, the phone rang, Ivy picked it up, and it was Julia. The sisters began to talk. They talked about their husbands, the weather, their kids, about starting a new public relations business, about roast chicken, about everything and nothing. Nothing at all to do with surrogacy. And that's how they knew they would be all right.

"Mama come here," says Ben as he crawls through the plastic play tunnel in the front yard. Julia pads down the stairs after her blond-haired boy and bends her long body into the hole. Ivy sits rocking on the wicker rocker on the porch, watching. In the beginning, Ivy had to fight the urge to throw herself all over him or to tell Julia how to raise him, feed him, mother him. She still works hard on giving them space. Ben is her nephew, and his mother is Julia. Her sister Julia. Her wisecracking, one-upping sister, the one Ivy brought back. As evening draws on, the sisters begin tossing one-liners over the fence, commenting to passersby, laughing at each other's jokes, loving each other's children. A family, by all appearances, like any other. All the relationships going forward are also always going back.

15 *A Hard Frost*

*H*ere's a gardening tip. When your life starts going south, put on your gloves and get on your knees and start praying. Pray for the beans to come up and the tomatoes to ripen, for the roses to take and the rhododendrons to bloom. Pray for good rain, a warm summer, pray for the slugs to meet the salt. Carol never gave this advice to her clients, not formally anyway. After years as a family therapist, she knew that what helped people in crisis was communicating well, identifying what was happening in their lives and what they wanted to happen, and paying attention to the process of making it happen. Still, if her own experience was any indication, there was much to be said for kneeling in dirt.

Often after a stressful day, Carol would head to her backyard garden in the Pacific Northwest. Her husband, Steve, was more likely to head to his computer. They met years earlier counseling at the same center, and they married into the comfort of the things they had in common: a professional life, a strong work ethic, a measured view of the world. At that time, he was forty-two, she was thirty-one. She hoped someday to raise a child. Women friends and clients said giving birth was the best moment in their lives. Carol wanted that, certainly, but more than that, she wanted to know and love a child. Steve was less certain. He had spent more than a decade of his adulthood as a Roman Catholic priest and never dreamed he would marry, much less have kids. He knew that people had children for all sorts of unhealthy reasons: because they felt incomplete or unloved. But he saw there were many healthy reasons to want to parent, too. The desire to give of yourself, to influence a developing life, the desire to improve the world by bringing a good, loving person into it. Who doesn't want to change the world?

When Carol didn't get pregnant, she and Steve went to a doctor. Carol was told to take her temperature. Steve was told he had low sperm count. And from then on, the spotlight was on him. Steve did everything he could to take care of "his" problem.

Few people understand how difficult it is to produce a sperm sample in a room designed for a urology exam. Steve knows the challenge well. The doctor at the university medical center would suggest Steve change some habit or medication. Steve would make the change. Then, he'd have to produce another sample, month after month. One month his sperm count was fine, the next terrible. There was no apparent obstacle, no illness, and, by all accounts, no reason for the variability. He switched from briefs to boxer shorts on the theory that tighter underwear raised scrotal temperature and killed the sperm, a theory that's been all but debunked. He stopped drinking alcohol; his count did not improve. He started taking antihistamines—on his doctor's advice—and the count still didn't improve. Steve felt frustrated and guilty for being the source of their problem. The word *defective* kept coming to his mind. In a year of consultations at the clinic, though, no one ever inquired after or included his wife, Carol. As much as he felt responsible, she felt shut out.

Yet Steve felt more and more motivated. His efforts to become a father had been like opening an undiscovered door, the force of how badly he wanted to become a parent surprised everyone. He began researching infertility on the Internet and came across articles on how ICSI was being used with impressive results to overcome poor sperm counts, motility, and morphology. His doctor had heard of it, but made it sound about as easy as a moon landing. Steve kept reading. He came across our center's website, and when he saw the treatments offered, he wanted to know more. Our center's embryologists were doing ICSI every day of the week.

. . .

It is April 1996 when I first consult with Steve and Carol. She is just turning thirty-seven, and Steve is forty-seven. They'd been trying to have a baby for three and a half years. A review of their charts tells me her hormone levels, uterus, and fallopian tubes are normal. His sperm analyses are not.

Most men are entitled to have one lousy sample because of a fever or a late night or stress. I see that Steve's sperm counts fluctuate substantially, from very low numbers of 1 million per millimeter to 51 million. Counts of 20 million are considered normal. You can see why such unpredictability can make a spontaneous pregnancy very difficult to achieve. When there is that much variation in multiple sperm samples, at least part of what we're up against is a male factor. After a year of searching, doctors couldn't pinpoint the cause of Steve's production problem. My challenge is to help Steve and Carol get around it. I explain that we can overcome the variability with in vitro fertilization by using ICSI.

In the fourteen months before Carol and Steve came to San Francisco, we performed 254 ICSI procedures; by the time they arrived, one hundred women had already had ultrasound scans confirming they were pregnant. ICSI had the ability to remove sperm problems as a factor.

I tell Carol and Steve that, for a woman her age, we're looking at a 37 to 40 percent chance that they will take home a baby with one in vitro fertilization cycle. Carol's cycle begins in early summer. First, she begins the drugs to suppress her own hormonal system, and then the fertility drugs to stimulate her ovaries. The daily injections become a ritual for her and Steve. They come into the house after work, get the ice pack from the freezer and head into the family room where Steve lines up the medications to prepare her shots.

It isn't easy for her, or for him. He doesn't like the idea of hurting her. But they're resigned that this is what they need to do. They talk a lot these evenings about the cycle and how they're getting through it. Steve takes over organizing everything, and Carol feels grateful and cared for. Like many of my patients, this couple has found that the injections become almost an act of intimacy. Infertility often interferes with other attempts to feel close. Steve and Carol both felt a distance develop between them in the year he spent pursuing a solution alone.

When a couple realizes a fertility problem exists, sex can begin to feel mechanical and then extraneous. What's the point? Feelings of blame, inadequacy, and a loss of sexual identity can emerge. Patients talk about not feeling feminine or not like a real man. Such grief takes a toll on the healthiest of relationships. The fact that one person in the relationship has the diagnosed problem also creates an enormous strain. In some cultures or religions, it is acceptable to divorce a partner if he or she cannot have a child. One of the most rewarding points of my career was helping a Jewish Orthodox couple, Abraham and Ruth, to start the family that their Judaism exhorted them to do. They had tried for more than two decades. At one point, it would have been acceptable for Abraham to leave his wife. Out of archetypal duty, Ruth offered to leave, but her offer was turned down. After more than twenty years of assisted reproduction, their extraordinary devotion and persistence was rewarded with the conception they had yearned for: twin sons. I spoke to Ruth recently, and she said, "I still can't thank God enough. And I still don't believe it when I get up in morning and hear, 'Mommy, Mommy.' I feel I can walk on the street with my head up. When everyone asks if I have children, I can say, 'Yes, two.' It feels great." I think of this couple's extraordinary relationship, and it refuels my desire to continue in this field.

By the time Carol and Steve get from the Pacific Northwest to San Francisco for the egg retrieval, they are excited and expectant. They plan some side trips, pick some good restaurants, and stay with friends. It feels more like a mini vacation than a medical appointment. Early on the morning of June 25, we retrieve ten eggs—a somewhat lower response than I expected—but Carol and Steve are pleased. They're on their way. But the morning of the transfer, the news from the laboratory is tempered. Only half the eggs fertilized normally, a quarter fewer than we usually see with ICSI. The five embryos that result are not the range of quality we had hoped for either. Normally at least 10 percent of the embryos in a given cycle are top notch, with no blemishes or irregular cells. None of these embryos are perfect; all of them have some degree of fragmentation, and the shells around the eggs appear quite thick.

Picture a turtle egg. Its shell is soft, not calcified like a chicken egg, yet it's quite a tough membrane that the little turtle has to rupture in order to be born. The human embryo, once it begins dividing, also has to rupture a shell, a clear membrane that holds the cells together. The embryo must "hatch" in order for the blastocyst or trophoblast cells to be able to bond with the cells of the uterine lining. If the membrane doesn't rupture, a perfectly normal embryo may never implant.

A major problem all in vitro fertilization doctors face is the failure of most embryos to implant. One reason we suspect implantation is so poor in some women is that their embryo shell, the zona pellucida, is so thick and tough that the expanding embryo cannot "hatch." Older women seem to have tougher shells, suggesting age may have a considerable influence on the zona pellucida, but even younger women may produce thick zonas.

In the earlier days of IVF, we used to lacerate the membrane physically with a needle, but that traumatized the fertilized egg. Then we started digesting the whole shell with an enzyme. The problem with that was that the toughest part is the inner membrane, so you had to go all the way through and possibly damage the embryo. Now, we use assisted hatching. In the laboratory, an embryologist holds the embryo with a narrow suction pipette and blows a very weak acid solution against the shell. It reduces the thickness of the shell right where the cells of the embryos are and leaves a weak spot for the embryo to rupture through and implant. I recommend this procedure for patients over age thirty-eight who have had a failed IVF cycle, or whenever a woman's zonas are thick.

I believe assisted hatching should help Carol and Steve. But we also need to make a good decision about how many embryos to put back. In the best circumstances, transferring three to four healthy embryos to women under forty gives us the best chance of a pregnancy. Given Carol's age and the quality of the embryos, I think we should consider transferring five, understanding, of course, that there is a small risk of a major multiple pregnancy and that they would need to be able to consider reduction.

Carol is a cautious woman. The kind of woman who, before she ever tried to become pregnant, had herself tested for HIV, though she'd done almost nothing in her life to be at risk for it. She needs to think over what I have said, and I leave her and Steve alone for a few minutes to discuss how many they're comfortable transferring.

Infertility forces even cautious people to gamble. Although there is risk in everything we do, I am not, by nature, a gambler. My grandfather, Spiros Louverdis, was a gambler, a native of Cephalonia, Greece, who emigrated to South Africa in 1908. He made a fortune as a wholesale businessman and lost it gambling in Monte Carlo, a pattern he repeated throughout his life. He would pull up to my parochial school in a big black Chrysler sedan, a legend in a black suit and snap-brimmed fedora. But my mother, who lived through the loss of those fortunes, was not a gambler, nor was my father. We never even liked playing cards.

So it is quite strange to be in a profession that demands an almost daily dose of risk. I try to tell patients there is risk in everything we do, from the procedures to the pregnancy. I try to give them the space and time to decide which outcome will be acceptable for them, just as I'm doing now with Steve and Carol. My job is to try to synthesize the essence of their problem and give them my best estimate of their chances that a particular approach will work so they can make a decision and move forward.

Carol and Steve decide to transfer all five and we proceed.

When they return home, Carol puts a photo of the embryos just prior to transfer on the refrigerator. A few days later she is telling an office mate about how the week went. Quite unexpectedly, the woman asks how many embryos were transferred.

"Five," Carol answers. She immediately regrets it. The woman looks horrified, and Carol quickly tries to explain that the chances of even getting one baby are quite low. But the woman is seeing five babies. She sees Carol as someone who would risk having five babies. From then on, Carol and Steve are very careful about what they say and to whom.

Steve feels great about how it's going. Carol is not a pessimist, but she finds herself taking each day as it comes, waiting for what seems an eternity to get the results. On July 7, she gets them.

"I'm sorry," the nurse says. "The results tell us that you are not pregnant at this time. Stop all medication. Expect a heavy period in seven to ten days. Schedule an appointment to speak to the doctor. A counselor is available. . . ."

Steve is stunned. This was it. ICSI was the answer. How could it not work? He is walking around in disbelief. Carol is filled with sadness. She gets up and goes out to the garden.

She spends the summer on her knees in the dirt. She digs up bushes, clears space for a deck, tears up the lawn, puts in a waterfall, plants perennials and two dozen rose bushes. She plants beans, peas, tomatoes, and basil. She coaxes the corn along. The corn isn't coming up.

They want to try again right away, but I tell them it's best to wait at least six to eight weeks. It takes at least a month for the ovaries to rest and recover from the stimulation. Emotionally, couples need time to acknowledge their loss. When a cycle fails, the casualties are multiple. There is the loss of the embryos, the loss of a potential baby, of all the time and the money invested. It is, for many people, a death, and they move through the stages of grief from denial to acceptance.

In September, when the vines are heavy with squash and the tomatoes fat, Carol and Steve come back to the city from the Northwest. We know we still are dealing with a male factor, but there seems to be a subtle egg problem, as well. Carol is thirty-seven, and blood tests tell us that she should respond a certain way to the ovulation drugs, but she doesn't. For this cycle, we decide to adjust her fertility drugs to try to get more and better eggs and, thus, a greater chance for good embryos. We're trying to win this numbers game by upping our percentages. In this attempt, we do get more follicles and more fertilization of the eggs using ICSI. The quality of the embryos improves, too, but just barely. We have eight embryos of average quality.

Here's what we need to consider, I tell them on the morning of the transfer. When we look at the variables, we're pulling every lever except numbers. We've had Carol taking heparin and aspirin in the last two cycles to overcome any possible antibody that may interfere with implantation. We are using every method in the laboratory to improve chances. We have one failed cycle behind us. The only other variable we can manipulate over last time is numbers. It's a tough line we walk. We want to give people the best chance of having a baby; we want to be aggressive, understanding that a couple can do selective reduction in the event of a major multiple. We discuss transferring all eight.

Steve has a momentary flash of the Dionne quintuplets plus three, but it doesn't linger. The chances of their having three or four implant sounds infinitesimally small. They know they're willing to do what it takes to have a baby. Together we agree to use all eight.

At home, in late September, the results of the pregnancy tests come in, and this time Carol and Steve cannot believe it. They did everything right, everything possible. The results are negative.

In a garden, the constant cold of winter does less damage than a hard frost in early autumn or late spring. A hard frost in September, when there is still good growing, will split bark and snap branches. It breaks evergreens. The plants are unprepared.

That fall, Steve withdraws. He works more, talks less, and generally feels pissed off. He cannot believe how many people complain about their children or mistreat them. No one else has a clue about what he is going through, not the grief, or the disappointment, or the cost.

The depression Carol feels descend isn't some icy blackness as much as it is damp gray, like breathing through heavy wool. She feels overwhelmed by the smallest tasks; she can't finish paperwork, open bills, or return cards. She starts seeing a therapist. As she talks, her training, her autopilot, kicks in. Infertility is a life stress, she says. It's a loss, the first time someone young and healthy finds out there is something wrong with them. Infertility is personal, making an individual feel different and less than. For some people, the experience and the treatment can remind them of every major issue in their past. She's analyzing herself. She's trying to help herself.

New Year's Day, 1997, their garden is frozen to stillness, the trees twisted bare. Carol and Steve are in San Francisco again. They had purchased a plan that gives a 90 percent money-back guarantee for up to three IVF attempts. Steve is anxious and feels determined to get this right the third time. Most of Carol's hope died in September. Now she feels like she is going through the motions.

We've changed the fertility drug protocol. I'm hoping for a change in the results of the quality of the embryos. The results do change. They're worse. Under the microscope, the perfect embryo has four or more cells, equal in size and shape, without a blemish. The ten embryos we are looking at the morning of the transfer are overwhelmingly fragmented. They look like a cookie crushed with the bottom of a glass. We have now transferred fifteen embryos in two cycles without a pregnancy. And we are faced again with deciding how many to put back.

Carol knows that when she started on her first cycle of in vitro fertilization she was different, in a different place. But this whole journey, with its discussion of risk and chance and disappointments, has changed her and what she is willing to do. She is more daring than she'd ever dreamed. She is willing, in some part of her, to do anything to have a baby. Together, we again decide to transfer all ten.

They go home and days later learn that Carol is not pregnant. She feels disappointment—and relief. Relief at not having a multiple pregnancy. Relief that it's done.

Three days later I telephone Carol and Steve from San Francisco. It's a one-hour call. Steve wonders if this could be a laboratory problem. Whenever we have embryos of less-than-average quality, we always look at the conditions in the laboratory that day. Temperature, the media the embryos were held in, and the embryologists working are considered, along with other cases that were handled the same day and the same week for comparison. It's not impossible that it was a lab problem. But looking at our records, overall the embryos that day and week were better than average. We have the numbers that demonstrate this. I tell Steve and Carol that I think we can be fairly certain that we're dealing with an egg problem. What are their chances if they do it again? Steve asks.

At Carol's age, thirty-eight, there is a 40 percent chance of taking home a baby, I say. But on the basis of their previous cycles, I think their chance would be 25 percent. Yes, they could consider a surrogate, but the embryos would be the same, and the only advantage would be that the surrogate would not have had to undergo the retrieval that can alter the body chemistry and rev up the immune system.

Are they just unlucky? This is probably not bad luck, I say. I think there is an egg factor here that cuts our chances in half. Really, the only way around it is to look at egg donation. That's the only modality of treatment that will fundamentally alter their situation. It's a huge decision. They need to take some time to think about it. We say good-bye and hang up.

As much as we can analyze what happened to Carol and Steve and whether it's the egg or the sperm or the combination of the two, it's a failure for me. Technically, I couldn't help them. Some days in this job are good, and some days, like this one, are downright awful.

When I started in in vitro fertilization, 90 percent of the people who tried IVF failed. Now it's 50 percent. In spite of the successes, it never gets any easier to deliver bad news. I guess I can only hope that I've given patients who've had a failed cycle enough information to take the next step and enough space to respect how they feel about it. You're trying to give people every chance to have their own genetic child, but at a certain point you have to step back and say that maybe you're at least helping them move along to the next step.

Every single couple at this point is crushed. And some people are angry. They used to be a lot angrier. Since 1995, our center has offered IVF patients a shared risk, or refund program, that refunds all or most of a couple's fee if they do not become pregnant. Shared-risk or money-back guarantee programs have been sharply criticized by several leading reproductive doctors and the American Medical Association as being exploitive, misleading, and contrary to long-standing tradition against charging contingency fees for medical service.

Most people don't have insurance for IVF, and I believe these kinds of programs give patients a certain amount of insurance against the risk of failure. The Ethics Committee of the American Society for Reproductive Medicine found that such programs are ethically acceptable as long as patients are well informed of the criteria, the fact that it costs more to participate in such a program than it would to have a single IVF cycle, and that screening and drugs are not included. The committee concluded that the plans it examined, including ours, provided sufficient information for patients to make an informed decision. The ASRM Committee is most worried, and rightly so, that such arrangements can create a conflict of interest in that the clinic is likely to make decisions not in the best interest of the patient but to avoid paying the refund. The committee has found no such evidence that either danger has materialized. And committee members point out that every reproductive center in the country has incentives to make treatment decisions in order to have high enough success rates that future patients are attracted.

To me, the problem is that many couples have only the money for one or two cracks at IVF or other fertility treatments, and that is why I feel so strongly about being able to give their money back if we can't help them have a baby. Nobody likes having to give bad news and then have to say, "Look it didn't work, but why don't you come back next September and pay another $10,000." The guarantee is a legitimate service to my patients that addresses risk so that when an IVF cycle fails, the couple who has to cope with that loss doesn't lose all their money. They have the means to get on with their lives.

Postscript

Carol went back to the garden. It felt good to put her hands in the earth. After six months of grieving, her therapist suggested ways to help them know what to do next.

Carol and Steve had four options: 1) to not have children, 2) to try another IVF cycle using donor eggs, 3) to adopt domestically, and 4) to adopt internationally. The therapist suggested ranking these options in two ways: first, by which would be most comfortable, and second, by which was most likely to happen.

Carol saw clearly that egg donation was in last place, comfort-wise. She had no problem raising a child that wasn't genetically related. That wasn't the issue. The problem was the same one that had haunted her previous in vitro cycles: She was afraid of a multiple pregnancy. She was terrified of getting pregnant with triplets or more and of then facing the prospect of having to have an abortion, delivering premature babies, or having babies who may be disabled or die.

Steve was interested in egg donation, but the cost and success rates were discouraging; even with donor eggs, there was a 50 percent chance the cycle would fail.

Carol's first choice was domestic adoption. In their relationship, Steve had always been the mover and shaker, Carol was the one in the garden, putting down roots. But on this matter she moved. She arranged a home study in August and an interview with an adoption facilitator in September. The interview occurred nearly a year, practically to the day, since the in vitro cycle in which Carol began to lose hope of ever having a child. The facilitator had in her purse information she had just received on a young mother looking for a family to adopt her baby. The facilitator asked if Carol and Steve would be interested in putting together a photo album and a letter to the prospective birth mother. They did it in three hours that night.

It wasn't that great a letter, but they addressed the birth mother by her first name and later learned that's what caught her eye. They enclosed photos of their cat. The birth mother, who was just twelve years old, was considering six interested couples. She wanted to meet Steve and Carol.

Carol and Steve were nervous. That week they met the birth mother, Cassie, and her mother, and her mother's boyfriend. They were two families from two different worlds. Steve and Carol then left on a scheduled vacation to Italy. When they returned, they learned Cassie had picked another couple. It was disheartening.

Steve said he didn't think he could get back on the roller coaster. He felt adoption offered the same kind of hopeful expectation followed by devastating failure that he and Carol had experienced through in vitro. The rejection, like the physiological barriers to pregnancy, was personal.

But then, Cassie changed her mind. She wanted to meet them again. They met the next day, a Saturday, at the mall, where they talked as they walked around. Cassie asked Steve and Carol who would take care of the baby during the day, and they said, "We both will." They planned to both work part-time and not use day care. Carol called their plan "share care."

On Sunday, Cassie's mother called and said that her daughter had chosen them. Three days later, on Wednesday afternoon, Carol was with a client when she got the call that Cassie was in labor. Carol drove fifty miles to the hospital, stopping to pick up the girl's family along the way. The girl was moved to another better-equipped hospital and given medicine to stop her labor. After a test showed the baby's lungs were sufficiently developed, she delivered.

The baby was a boy, born that Friday. Just five days after Carol and Steve learned that they were going to become parents, they were holding their son in their arms.

Cassie visits their home twice a year, and when she and her family arrive, it is clear that they see Carol and Steve as the parents. Carol says she has learned that the key is flexibility, of never saying never, as in, "I would never tolerate an open adoption." Their experience has not been at all threatening.

Sometimes Steve gets the ghost, the sense he would have liked to have had a genetic child of his own, but then he realizes that he and Carol could not have asked for a more wonderful or better-natured boy than the one they are raising. They savor their son. They have, to this day, an appreciation for the process of pregnancy and childbirth, a sense of awe. From the first in vitro cycle, they have been amazed that anyone gets pregnant. They don't regret they tried in vitro fertilization, but they feel cautioned by it.

"When you go to the doctor and get medication, you expect to be cured, and in this, 30 percent are cured," Steve said. "We did everything we were supposed to do, and it didn't work. I think you have to go in with your eyes open. I wish we had talked to another couple ourselves beforehand so that we understood that better going in."

The photos of embryos that once were taped to their refrigerator door have been replaced by photos of a laughing baby. Carol no longer visits Internet infertility chat rooms or remembers many of the details from that period of her life, just two years earlier. When she goes into the garden, she cannot believe how many poisonous plants are out there. They're coming out. When she gets the time.

"Having a child made all the difference," she says.

16 Survivors

$\mathcal{A}$nne was at an infertility workshop to learn about egg donation and surrogacy when she realized the experts onstage could be talking about her.

Her hand shot up. "I've had breast cancer, and I'm menopausal. Could I carry a baby?"

"Yes," the doctors said.

"Could I breast-feed?"

"Probably."

For the first time in years, Anne has hope of becoming a mother. She was thirty-seven when a small, firm mass in her left breast made her the first case of breast cancer in her family. She underwent a lumpectomy, five weeks of radiation, and a year of chemotherapy drugs injected into the veins on the back of her hand every Tuesday. She swallowed capsules of cyclophosphamide (Cytoxan) and prednisone, endured injections of methotrexate, 5-fluorouracil, and vincristine. Her oncologist warned that the treatment might precipitate her into premature ovarian failure.

Toward the end of her chemotherapy, Anne would be sitting at her desk in a federal office and feel a surge of warmth, her skin turning bright red, her brow running with rivulets of sweat. Hot flashes signaling the menopause. "My own personal summer," she'd say.

The timing was cruel. Anne was the oldest of eight, and she wanted children. She'd waited to start a family so her husband, Warren, could finish a book he'd been researching and writing for a decade. The week she started chemotherapy, they celebrated the book's completion. Now that they were ready to have children, physically she no longer could. Anne wondered if she'd had children earlier in her life, as her sisters had, whether she might have avoided the breast cancer all together. She wondered too, if there was more to life than this. She had supported her husband since they married, working through her treatment, even as the weekly chemical assaults ground her to a frail exhaustion. At year's end, Warren still hadn't gotten a job or sold his book. They couldn't afford a car for her, couldn't travel or go to concerts or go out to dinner or do anything that might make life without children tolerable for her. Anne was angry and tired of being broke and joyless. She packed and left.

"I want a bigger life," she told a friend. "A fuller life."

A year later, Anne volunteered at one of the largest state parks in California, where in five minutes she could be on a hiking trail where she wouldn't see anyone. She'd been a bird-watcher for years; it was one of the few hobbies she could afford during her first marriage, and she loved being outdoors. She studied wildflowers and trail systems and the birds of Northern California. One night another park volunteer followed her to the parking lot and asked her to dinner. Nick was a tall, athletic, electrical engineer who'd been involved in serious relationships before, but had never been married. On their first date, they drove to the Marin headlands to count the migrating hawks and see the raptors, then into the city for dinner. He asked her if she wanted to have children. His number one priority, he said, was to get married and have kids.

"Sorry. You don't want to go out with me then," she said, and surprising herself, began to cry. She told him about the cancer and what the treatment had done. Nick asked why she couldn't have children through assisted reproduction. She told him it was a door she was reluctant to open. After the cancer, she grieved the loss of her fertility; it was devastating, but she had moved on. Revisiting that emotional turmoil, especially since the technology could fail, seemed inordinately risky, she explained.

Nick took risks. He'd changed careers four times since college and, for relaxation, skied downhill and flew gliders. Once they began seriously to see each other, he'd drive to Stanford University to research in vitro fertilization, excited by the leaps in technology that were being made: intracytoplasmic sperm injection, embryo adoption. Buoyed by his enthusiasm, the couple joined the national infertility support group RESOLVE. Anne's mother and sisters were thrilled at this new man in Anne's life, who was so committed to having a family and so able to help Anne see the possibilities in assisted reproduction.

Anne's younger sister, Maggie, an accountant and the mother of two, offered to donate her eggs. Her sister-in-law offered to be the gestational surrogate and carry their child. And that was how "the team of four" wound up at a weekend workshop on different approaches to infertility. That was when Anne first learned *she* could carry a child; a carefully choreographed schedule of hormones could help her get—and stay—pregnant.

"That's what I want to do," she told Nick.

They arrive at my office on a crisp autumn afternoon. San Francisco Bay glistens in the sunshine. Anne watches a flock of birds fly in a wide V off to the west. She flips through a photo album in the waiting room. There are, she notices, a lot of twins.

When I meet them for the first time, I think they are a striking couple. She is clearly a survivor and crystal clear in what she wants to do. Nick seems very intense and focused. They had gone to one of our fertility seminars a few months earlier, and I remembered them sitting in the front row. Anne had gone through menopause nearly six years before because of her chemotherapy. She is forty-two.

Most cancer treatment can affect a woman's ability to have children temporarily, and, in some cases, permanently. Chemotherapy drugs can damage the genetic material in eggs or precipitate a full menopause. Bone marrow transplants almost always cause permanent ovarian damage. Surgery and radiation, especially of the pelvis, can cause scarring of the fallopian tubes, uterus, and vagina. Radiation can damage the hypothalamus and pituitary gland.

Men with cancer are also affected, either by direct damage of the testicle or damage to the ejaculation mechanics. But for more than twenty years men have been able easily to bank their sperm before their treatment begins, while the practice of egg freezing is just starting.

Until recently, there was no option for women to bank eggs. We had only the technology to freeze an egg already fertilized that had grown into an embryo, using techniques that had been developed by Dr. Alan Trounson and his team in Australia in 1984. Freezing women's eggs is a process just emerging; for years success was elusive. At the time of her illness, Anne's only option was to freeze her embryos, but when she looked into that before her treatment, the cost for her one-income family seemed prohibitively expensive.

Many times people regret what they did or did not do in regard to their fertility. Decisions to use birth control, postpone childbearing, terminate an unplanned pregnancy, or, in this case, face the simple inability to afford the procedures, can cause people to second-guess decisions they made years earlier. As if the stress of infertility isn't enough, many people I treat wrestle with guilt and a constant feeling of "what if?" But we all make decisions in our lives, and, in that space in time, we must conclude that they were the right ones. We made that decision with the information available to us at the time. We need to forgive ourselves for trying to do the right thing.

I think back on my own life, and there was a time, in my mid-thirties, after my first marriage ended in divorce, that I never thought I'd ever have a family of my own. I remember telling my mother and stepfather, Louis, that it was so strange that I was working to help all these families to have babies when I didn't have any prospects myself. I understand what Anne must have been feeling all these years, and how meeting Nick was, for her, like meeting Miriam was for me, a new beginning, a second chance.

Anne will obviously require an egg donor. Many other conditions also require egg donation, including premature ovarian failure either from cancer treatment or a chromosomal disorder like Turner's syndrome, and unexplained ovarian failure associated with autoimmune diseases. Although she had once considered it her only option, Anne does not want to use a surrogate. "It may not be my genetic child, but at least if I can carry it, I can be part of it. If it's my sister's eggs in my sister-in-law's body, it feels too removed."

For the first time, Nick balks. He knows it can be dangerous for a survivor of breast cancer, a hormone-dependent cancer, to risk the hormonal storm of pregnancy. And his concern is absolutely warranted.

The woman before me survived cancer, a major life crisis. Anne's disease has been treated, and we have the technology to help her become pregnant with her sister's eggs. But the biggest question we face is: How will this affect Anne's health?

I cannot accept a cancer survivor for treatment without her oncologist's approval. It is vital that the oncologist be involved. First, because the patient needs to continue to be monitored by her caregiver, but also, if there is a recurrence of cancer, the oncologist is then already in the loop.

Anne's oncologist is cautious, but gives his permission. "I've come to realize you're going to do what you want to do," he tells Anne. They've known each other since her original diagnosis. She sees him at her checkup every six months. He knows she's a strong-willed woman and how badly she wants a child. The American Society of Reproductive Medicine states that the survival of most cancer patients is not affected by subsequent pregnancy.

Nick agrees to try to have a child with Anne using donated eggs. Many women go with an anonymous donor who is under age thirty-five. Anne wants to use the eggs of her younger sister, Maggie, who is thirty-six. Nick feels a lot is riding on the process. He wants children so badly that if they can't have them together, he can't promise the relationship will last. These are the words anyone who is infertile fears most: the fear of being left as damaged goods.

Nick tries to explain this statement, which he knows is deeply wounding for Anne. He's trying to be as honest as possible in saying that, as an only child himself and then as a single adult, he's almost never held a baby. He wants to father, to bring his own genetic children into the world. It's a life experience that he doesn't want to miss.

Anne takes a hard-eyed look into the future and sees that, if they pursue in vitro fertilization and it fails, she'll be broke, devastated, and then dumped by her boyfriend. Nope, she says evenly. Either you're with me because you love me and want to be with me, with or without children, or you're not. If you're not, there is no sense going any further. "We're going to be together long after the kids," she says.

It was true, he realizes. They love each other, and he knows that finding the right person is a rare thing. They decide to get married in the spring. But, given Anne's and Maggie's ages, they don't want to wait until then to begin a cycle.

In October, they start the medication. With six years and four other siblings separating them, Anne and Maggie weren't that close as kids. In the months to come, they will grow very close.

The couple never formally ask for Maggie's help; they don't have to. She is overjoyed with the prospect.

"This is an amazing thing to be able to give to somebody," Maggie tells her husband. "It's incredible."

Now that we've made the decision to proceed, the next step is to synchronize and then begin the two women's cycles. Anne and Maggie are both a little surprised at how preoccupied they feel about the regimen and how much time they spend talking about it on the phone. Both women work, and they managed to arrange ultrasounds and blood tests either before or after work or on weekends and holidays.

The night before the retrieval, Maggie stays at Nick and Anne's house while her husband is at home with their two small children. Nick and Anne are upbeat, making family plans for the coming holidays. Shops and offices are already putting up Christmas decorations, and it isn't even Thanksgiving. On November 18, Maggie comes in for the retrieval. She responds well to the drugs and produces twenty-four eggs. She feels a little giddy, like a teenager. The eggs are mixed with Nick's sperm.

Three days later, as Anne and Nick drive into the city for the transfer, Anne is pensive.

"This is probably the happiest we'll be for a while," she says quietly. "We have all these hopes that this will work." At the conference before the transfer, the news from the laboratory is not good. Only eleven of the eggs fertilized. None of the embryos are perfect. Three are graded as good, but the rest are of poor grade, with many fragments and irregular cells. The lining of Anne's uterus is also of less than optimal thickness.

Given this news, our meeting is solemn. Considering the compromised quality of the embryos, we'll have to transfer a larger number to have any chance of even a single embryo implanting. I tell this to Anne and Nick. We agree to transfer all eleven, understanding that we run a risk of a major multiple pregnancy that may require selective reduction. The transfer goes smoothly. An hour later, the couple leaves my office and walk five blocks to Fisherman's Wharf for lunch.

Ten days later, the couple go to the clinic for the pregnancy test, and, as they walk back into the kitchen upon returning home, they see the light blinking on their answering machine. They had asked the staff to call with the pregnancy results immediately, even if the nurse had to leave the results on the recorder. They hit "play."

"You are not pregnant at this time," says the nurse's voice on the tape. The anguish Anne fears most is now a reality. Nick shakes his head, thinking, What's the next step? Crying, Anne picks up the phone to call Maggie.

Maggie is devastated by how few of the eggs fertilized and how few became good-quality embryos. She is healthy and young; she has children. What is wrong with me? she asks herself. "I'd been on a high, thinking that I produced eggs like a teenager, when I saw that, in reality, they were faulty. I thought, oh my God," she says.

Three weeks later, on a gloomy December day, Anne and Nick and I speak in a conference at the office. The question is, Why didn't it work?

Let's look at the variables: the eggs, the embryos, the lining of the uterus, and the immunology. Normally, 70 percent of mature eggs fertilize. Less than 50 percent of Maggie's eggs did. There may have been a problem with the sperm attaching to the egg, or some of the eggs may not have been as mature as they should have been, given the stimulation and ripening of the follicles. There are techniques to help overcome those issues, I say. We can perform ICSI, which gives us more information about maturity of the egg and overcomes any egg-sperm interaction problem. We can double the amount of estrogen by injection and add a vaginal suppository to help boost the lining of Anne's uterus. But I point out that no matter how plump the lining is, we are still using nearly thirty-seven-year-old eggs.

I tell Anne and Nick that they might want to consider a younger donor. As much as the laboratory and the hormones are important, the single biggest factor in a successful cycle is the age of the egg. Choosing another, unrelated donor is a huge decision, which brings up the other options the couple has, of either adopting or remaining child-free. This is not a decision that can and should be made immediately. They say they'll call me back.

On the drive home, Anne and Nick decide to consider a younger anonymous donor. Anne makes an appointment at the donor agency. She goes into the city alone, circles the block twice looking for parking. Once inside, she takes a seat at a table in a small private room, and opens the first of five fat black binders before her. She reads page after page of profiles of young women. One thing she can't help noticing: None of them has red hair.

Anne realizes at this point that she needs to try one more cycle with Maggie. The red hair, the highlights, strawberry streaks, whatever it is that runs through her mother and her sisters' hair, she connects it to her family's uniqueness, and the tie to the people she loves the most.

Maggie is thrilled to try again—as soon as possible. When they notify me, I'm already planning for our laboratory to do ICSI. I believe the technique may overcome a problem that the sperm may have attaching to the egg. Second, because the eggs are peeled before the procedure, the laboratory staff can identify exactly how many eggs are mature rather than assuming most are. We are also going to use assisted hatching just prior to embryo transfer. I recommend assisted hatching for all eggs thirty-eight years or older, or for all patients with a previous failed IVF cycle and for all embryos with shells thicker than 15 microns.

It is winter in the Bay when Maggie, Anne, and Nick start the second cycle, and the drive home from work is usually in the dark. In their daily phone calls, Anne and Maggie agree that the first cycle felt so daunting, this one already feels easier. The sisters have their injection schedules down pat. On the day of the egg retrieval, they are both calm and ready.

They had spent several weeks strategizing about ways to reduce Anne's stress after the transfer. For this cycle I had decided to increase Maggie's stimulation protocol, and I'm able to retrieve seventeen eggs; three days later, after the eggs are fertilized and cultured, there is a modest improvement in embryo quality from the last cycle, with four good- and six poor-quality embryos.

Considering the bitter disappointment of the previous cycle, and understanding that with our decision comes the risk of multiple pregnancies, we agree to transfer the best eight embryos.

After Anne rests for the required hour after the transfer, she and her husband meet with a nurse who instructs them on the medication and a list of dos and don'ts. As Anne and Nick leave, the nurse tells them to think positive, "You are pregnant."

Anne believes him. She believes that after the last transfer, it was a mistake to go to lunch and back to work the following day. This time she goes home and straight to bed. She lies down with a stack of videos and magazines, and relaxes for ten days. When the results of the pregnancy test are telephoned to her house ten days after the transfer, Nick is off gliding. He finds a note when he returns: "Gone to get prenatal vitamins. We're pregnant!"

She calls Maggie, crying. "We're pregnant."

"Put your feet up!" Maggie shrieks. "We're pregnant!"

As it turns out, Anne is pregnant with twins.

Postscript

Anne and Nick had agreed that, because their egg donor was over thirty-five, they would undergo amniocentesis, in which the amniotic fluid is extracted, and the cells shed by the growing fetus are cultured and examined for genetic defects such as Down's syndrome. But when the time came to have the procedure, Anne refused to do it.

"I have put so much effort into getting pregnant. What am I going to do if there is a problem?" she said. "I'm not going to terminate." Nick was upset, but he accepted her position.

The couple married at Monterey Bay in early June, when she was four months along. The weather was perfect, and her floor-length gown didn't betray her condition, although the dozens of buttons down the back would likely not have closed just two weeks later. The minister made a special point of thanking Maggie. The happy couple and their guests ate tiramisu wedding cake and danced. It was a magical day.

Anne didn't enjoy being pregnant. Her sense of smell was so acute that working in a large office, where several people wore some fragrance or other, was difficult. Her ankles also swelled so much that she had trouble wearing shoes after her seventh month.

She was talking to Maggie on the phone at about thirty-seven weeks when she said, "I think I just wet my pants."

"Call the doctor and call Nick at work," Maggie said. "Your water just broke."

The following day, just after noon, Anne delivered twins, a boy, James, and a girl, Rose, healthy and normal, weighing over four pounds apiece. "A dream come true," she said. She had wanted two.

For Anne and Nick, starting a marriage and having two infants in the same year wasn't easy. Caring for two babies was exhausting. The babies were up all night and on different schedules. Nick and Anne were on different schedules, as well. Nick was a night owl, she was a lark. They started going to counseling to learn to find middle ground.

Maggie returned to her life, which was busy with her husband, children, and work. She said, "People think I should feel a real serious connection to Anne's babies. I do. But I don't feel they're my babies. They're Anne and Nick's babies. Anne carried twins; she created beautiful and perfect babies. She and Nick are wonderful parents. I'm ecstatic that I have been able to help."

Both women plan on telling their children about the conception when they're old enough to understand. But they don't really speak of their experience outside of the family.

Anne used to wonder sometimes why she survived the cancer when a good friend who was fighting at the same time didn't. She doesn't wonder anymore. The twins consume, absorb, and enliven her. "The medical thing is such a small part of it. It fades away as you go through life with your children."

She has a new circle of friends, mothers of twins. They are nine women, mostly older moms, who live within seven miles of one another and whose children all were conceived, coincidentally, with medical assistance and most by in vitro fertilization. They have a play group that gathers weekly and the mothers talk about the demands of motherhood, about diapers and breast-feeding. Anne breast-fed both twins for seven months on her healthy breast.

"The human body is a miraculous thing," she says.

17　Two Mothers

*I*n the Philippines, there is a child's game called pabitin, in which toys hang from strings attached to a colorful frame overhead and children take turns leaping and jumping toward the dangling treasures, pulling and knocking them down. It is a piece of perfect childhood, the Mexican piñata meets Christmas. Ginny's favorite.

Ginny remembers the game and the laughter and her mother, like shorn string, just out of reach.

She was born in a small city outside Manila, into a family of prominence and means. She lived on an estate, a legacy from her maternal grandfather, with her father, her mother, and younger sister. Next door lived the twenty-two-year-old cousin who one night took a pool stick and beat Ginny's mother to death, shot her only sister to death, then shot Ginny, too.

Ginny was fourteen. She awoke in a hospital days later, wounded in her head by her cousin's drug-crazed attempt to capture their inheritance. A month later, the gouges under Ginny's thick, black hair healed, her father asked her teacher, a Catholic nun, to reveal the news. It was then that Ginny was told her mother and sister were dead. Her mother was a gentle woman who had stopped working to be home with her daughters. Ginny's sister had been her playmate and confidante since birth.

By year's end, Ginny's father had married again and started a second family. Ginny crept quietly to the family's edge. She finished high school and went to college to study liberal arts and psychology. One day she came to the United States on holiday. While visiting her father's friends from their hometown in the Philippines, she met Raye.

She had never met anyone like her. Raye was a solar system, people were drawn to her, warmed by her. She was ambitious, accomplished in the insurance business, and, despite being from Ginny's hometown, very American. She drove fast and had a deep, infectious laugh.

Raye also remembered the murders well. Like everyone else in their hometown, she had gone to the funerals while Ginny was still in the hospital, unaware of the tragedy.

It was strange for Ginny to meet, years later and in the United States, this woman who knew so much about her. Within days, they felt intensely and mystifying close to each other. When Ginny returned home to the Philippines, she and Raye had long phone conversations for the next year. At that point, Ginny felt safe enough to step past all the warnings of her father and the Catholic church and her own preconceived image of the future, and into an elopement eventually formalized into a domestic partnership in downtown San Francisco. They were happy. Over the years, Raye's parents came to look at Ginny as "the daughter we never had."

"What about me?" Raye would say with mock outrage. Since she was six, she rejected her gender role, dressing like a son, playing like a son. By college Raye knew she was gay, and she also understood that she must leave the Philippines and her small, close-knit family to explore what that meant. Still, she was the only daughter, and she wanted her parents to have grandchildren.

Ginny had dreamed of having children her whole life. Seeing other couple's children, watching families grow around her, made her life feel empty. Ginny had talked to Raye about having artificial insemination or involving a friend, but it all seemed so unlikely to her. One morning she saw a doctor discussing in vitro fertilization on television, explaining egg and sperm donation, and suddenly she knew what was possible. She could see them having the children they both wanted—together.

.   .   .

Ginny and Raye are nervous in the elevator rising to our fifth-floor offices, unsure of the reception that two women will receive. In the waiting room, Ginny stands before the panoramic windows looking out on San Francisco Bay. To the west stands the weathered walls of Alcatraz, the notorious island prison that draws a million visitors a year. In the Philippines, Ginny's cousin served twelve years for the murders of her mother and sister, she thinks as she sees the prison. But her sentence seems ongoing. The murders took her family from her childhood, and also took it from her adulthood. The loss she felt at fourteen would feel even greater at thirty. It was cumulative.

Ginny doesn't work outside the home. When she looks at the high-rise buildings in the city around her, she envisions herself trapped in an elevator with a killer. It quiets a lot of ambition. She manages investments from a home office, takes cares of their one-bedroom apartment, and takes care of Raye. But Ginny is shy and withdrawn even with friends. In the car culture of California, she has never gotten a driver's license. Raye can't believe that Ginny's propelled them here.

According to their histories, Ginny's ovaries and uterus are in excellent health. Raye's are, too. They ask me if it's possible for gay partners to undergo in vitro fertilization. They want to conceive using Raye's egg, a sperm donor, and Ginny's body.

They have no gay friends who are parents. They have almost no gay friends. Their circle is a tight radius of extended family and close friends from work, all straight and married, all with children. They've wanted a child a long time. They use the prospective name as their computer passwords and bank card PINs for ten years. In their dreams, the child is Raelin, a girl.

Family is the basic unit of Filipino culture, each person part of a circle of extended relations. The circle grows through marriage and ritual coparenthood, the Catholic tradition of naming godparents who become as important as kin. Raye and Ginny are godparents five times over. "We have so much love to give," Raye says.

They are nervous. Almost immediately I suspect that Ginny had survived some significant trauma, there is something about her that is very fragile. I want them to feel very comfortable about being here. I have helped many same-sex couples before; the pregnancy rate is extremely high, given that these couples usually are infertile by circumstance rather than as a result of any organic pelvic disease.

Thirty years ago on the streets outside my office, sailors embarking in San Francisco beat gays without compunction. Fortunately, much of society's attitude has changed and acceptance has increased. Eight million gays and lesbians are parents in the United States; the majority are raising children from earlier heterosexual relationships. More recently, same-sex couples have begun creating families of their own through in vitro fertilization, surrogacy, and sperm donation.

I tell Ginny and Raye that many couples who share their circumstances have come to our center with dreams and left with children. This makes many people uncomfortable. The primary political opposition to recognizing marriages between gays and lesbians in the United States is based on the fear that gay couples will then become parents. In several countries, such as Denmark, gays are barred from receiving assisted reproduction in public clinics. Nontraditional couples enjoy far less of the traditional protection of family law.

At our clinic, we do not discriminate or withhold services on the basis of sexual orientation, age, or marital status. When we face issues like these, as well as complicated individual cases, we rely on the advice and direction of our own specially constituted ethics advisory board. The four men and women who serve are available to review broad ethical issues as well as individual patients.

Fertility doctors must constantly evaluate competing rights: the rights of the patient, the rights of the unborn child, the rights of society, and the rights of third parties such as sperm and egg donors and surrogates. The physician's primary responsibility is to the couple seeking medical intervention. Physicians cannot be the gatekeepers of social morality. We are hoping to help caring, committed people have families.

Should fertility physicians be forced to morally judge the ability of all couples who present for treatment on their suitability to parent? Some people feel it is the physician's responsibility. Yet society does not attempt to regulate the suitability of other adults—and even adolescents—who do not require assisted reproduction.

What is the impact of having gay parents? I don't know. In a survey of more than forty studies, the American Psychological Association concluded that the children of gay parents are as well adjusted as other children, and have similar IQs, play experiences, friendships, and sense of sexual identity. Other small and controversial studies show that the gay parents have a higher percentage of children who later turn out gay themselves than straight parents do. Some researchers, who believe homosexuality is largely genetic, say that makes sense. The studies will continue.

As a society, a far more troubling ethical dilemma is practically upon us. The advance of genetics, or, should I say, eugenics, may lead to a time when embryos can be screened for a predisposition to being gay or short or fat or redheaded. When will being different become undesirable? This is the real dilemma that we must confront. But it must be addressed by society, the law, and ethicists, and not solely by individual physicians acting as morality police.

Quite apart from Raye and Ginny being a same-sex couple, I have a medical concern about their situation. There may be less expensive and less invasive options available to them. Have they considered undergoing artificial insemination with donated sperm? The procedure, provided by a number of clinics in the Bay area, is minimally invasive and a fraction of the cost.

"We both want to be part of the child," Raye says.

I tell them that involving both of them will require two sets of medical tests, the coordination of two body clocks, and the administration of drugs to both.

"We both want to be involved," Raye says again.

Only when the nurses describe the clinic's protocol does she balk. Raye hates needles and is worried about the injections.

"Be motivated! If you really want to have a baby, to be a mother, you have to be motivated," Ginny says.

The women have already decided that Ginny wants to carry the pregnancy. She is the quintessential nurturer, wanting to make a home for her children and her partner.

Our challenge is to synchronize their menstrual cycles, stimulate Raye's ovaries, and prepare Ginny's uterus to receive the eggs fertilized by a sperm donor. A frozen sperm sample will be thawed the morning of the transfer. Although freezing can damage up to 50 percent of the sperm in a sample, we are still left with enough to fertilize eggs.

Some couples ask a friend or a family member to donate sperm. Raye and Ginny considered it—they have many good male friends—

but they worry that it may raise legal and psychological paternity issues in the future. This child already has two parents—why should they further complicate the situation. An anonymous donor makes more sense.

When Ginny and Raye contact a sperm bank they already have a type of donor in mind. They want a man with French heritage, in large part because a friend's French-Asian child is so gorgeous. The sperm bank they choose does not share donor pictures, so they narrow the list of candidates to three by comparing the medical histories, hobbies, and education of different men. Finally, they select a student at the University of California Los Angeles. He has a 4.0 grade point average, is over six feet tall, and musically inclined. He is twenty-two years old and French.

Now we are ready to proceed. I've instructed both women to start the birth control pill. Despite many years of living together, they have almost never had their periods at the same time because Raye is irregular. Ginny prepares their daily shots and administers all the injections, giving Raye Lupron to prevent unwanted ovulation and then stimulating drugs to affect her follicles. After seven days of taking fertility medication, Raye begins to leave her office at noon to undergo a daily blood test and ultrasound to monitor the follicular development. The couple is excited and open with their friends. Raye shares with her boss the purpose of her midday comings and goings.

His only question is, "What does that cost?"

When tests indicate that Raye's follicles are mature, Ginny administers her hCG shot at the appointed time, triggering the final maturation of the eggs. The retrieval is a success. Raye, thirty-four, has produced twenty-two eggs. I routinely order ICSI when using frozen sperm to avoid being surprised by a massive die-off at the time of thaw. Four days before Christmas, we learn from the laboratory that twenty-one of the eggs fertilized. Of the resulting embryos, fourteen are flawless. We decide to transfer six. The couple opts to freeze and store the remainder for a future cycle. Raye and Ginny don't expect this to work the first time.

After the transfer, they consult with the nurse, who instructs them on the medication and appointments for the coming weeks. The nurse says as they leave, "Keep in mind that you are pregnant."

Raye immediately starts talking to Ginny's tummy.

Ten days later, it's New Year's Day. The commute across the Golden Gate Bridge is a dream, the city is still asleep, nursing a hangover. The clinic, though, is already buzzing with patients, phone calls, and appointments; the eggs and sperm are all blissfully unaware that it's a holiday. Ginny and Raye arrive early. This is the day that they learn whether their cycle is a success.

The level of pregnancy hormone in the blood is obvious and rising at a rate that suggests to me that Ginny is pregnant with more than one. The nurse telephones them that afternoon when the results come in. "Congratulations," she says. "The tests indicate you are pregnant at this time."

Late in the day, after everything is quieted down and just a few tasks and staff remain, I remembered how nervous Raye and Ginny were at their first visit. I pick up the telephone to call to congratulate them.

I hear voices and laughter in the background from the party they are having. After the nurse called, friends and relatives crowded into their apartment to salute Ginny, who is wearing a new blue dress—a maternity dress. They are so thrilled that I have to laugh and savor this for just a moment. When a family is so excited, and the process works as it should, I find that I have to pause and store a little bit of the psychic high to help me though the cases that are negative.

From that day on, Ginny is the baby maker. Raye takes over the cooking, the laundry, and housekeeping. She drives Ginny up to the doors of malls and banks, so she won't have to cross parking lots. She asks hopefully if Ginny is having any 2 A.M. cravings and is disappointed that Ginny apparently isn't.

The couple is so excited at the first ultrasound at six weeks that, when they see the flutter of three heartbeats on the monitor, there is a distinct and sobering double take. Three is a big number. One heartbeat appears fainter than the others and the sac smaller. I tell them that, on the basis of the difference in the size of the gestational sacs, there's a good chance the smallest one won't survive. Sometime in the next few days, the third embryo slips away.

On Valentine's Day, at ten weeks, an ultrasound shows two heartbeats. Each sac and fetus is measured and photographed individually. At the end of the procedure, I hand Raye a "family portrait," a printout in the shape of a heart.

Raye walks down the hallway showing nurses, laughing that wonderful laugh. "They both look like me," she says.

Postscript

That week Raye traded in their Acura for a minivan—with car seats and room for strollers. She moved them into a new two-bedroom condominium. Her enthusiasm was infectious.

But as the pregnancy progressed, Raye began having nightmares of the twins being born of different ethnic backgrounds as occurred to a Dutch couple in an in vitro fertilization scandal in December 1993. The woman's egg was mistakenly inseminated with her husband's sperm as well as that of a man from the Caribbean island of Aruba. The result was twins—one black, one white. Raye would wake up crying and sweating. Images of a blond-haired blue-eyed child and a French-Filipino child rose before her.

"These are your children, too," Ginny said quietly. "We have to love them no matter what."

Whenever scandal or unethical behavior is discovered among fertility centers, it unleashes a firestorm of fear, phone calls, and criticism throughout the field. Patients now have to worry that these things may have happened to their eggs and sperm, believing it's a common occurrence. In fact, these incidents are extremely rare. There are hundreds of thousands of in vitro cycles performed safely and ethically.

Yet Raye's reaction is perfectly understandable. How can the loss of control not be frightening when your gametes, the very bearers of your unique genetic message, are relinquished to a laboratory? When the union that usually happens in the privacy and sanctity of a couple's bedroom is in the hands of total strangers. The enormity of this transaction is always with me and my staff. The best fertility centers have policies and procedures in place to check and double-check the identity of gametes. At our center, each couple's gametes are tracked by the name of the egg provider with a cross reference when the sperm provider has a different name. We designate a specific location in the laboratory, and we use a buddy system so that each step of the process is witnessed by another embryologist, checked and double-checked by another set of eyes. In the case in the Netherlands, a laboratory worker reusing a pipette inadvertently carried the sperm from one family into the dish of another. The result was a set of twins with the same mother but two fathers.

I can only reassure worried patients like Raye that, in our center, all equipment that comes into direct contact with gametes is disposable to safeguard against this very occurrence. But tragic events like these should serve as a reminder to the entire field to redouble their efforts to protect families.

Unfortunately, in spite of these reassurances, Raye continued to worry. Ginny, though, was radiant. She gained fifty pounds. At the mall, strangers would ask to pat her tummy. "Twins! You look so good." She felt herself opening up, talking and telling people that she had conceived in vitro and was having the children with Raye. People reacted positively. She felt, for the first time, proud of who she was.

At 12:09 A.M. on a hot August night, Ginny delivered two six-pound baby boys—by C-section because they were both breech. When she heard the cries and saw their jet-black hair, she nearly collapsed. Raye's fears of a blond-haired, blue-eyed mix-up disappeared with the boys they named Gabe and Gabby.

"It's a miracle. A miracle."

At every juncture in the women's long relationship, Raye's parents asked them to meet with a Catholic priest for advice or, more pointedly, absolution. Raye had once considered joining the Carmelite sisters, and she remained close to several nuns. When she and Ginny moved in together and when they got pregnant, they did talk to a priest who, in both instances, offered support and prayers. They went to the priest again, this time to have the boys baptized.

"Where is your husband?" the priest asked.

Raye took a deep breath. "Before we go any further, this is going to be like a confession." She blurted out the story of their relationship, their high-tech conception, and the family they now had. "If there is a problem with us being here, we can leave," she offered.

"No, no," the priest said. He counseled them a long time and welcomed the boys to be baptized. He couldn't help asking, though, how much the procedure cost.

"A lot," Raye said with a laugh. "But I'm not telling you how much."

The twins were baptized in sunlight and lace on a Sunday morning, along with six other babies, their presence a unique seal of their parents' life together. Ginny found in Raye the love and security she had lost as a child and felt that in their children, she had rediscovered the future. She began opening up to other people, resumed driving lessons, and felt, at last, that her life was complete.

"This is more binding and more permanent and real than anything," Raye said. "We're a family."

In every way but one. Raye had no legal ties to the boys. Since the women were not legally married, Ginny was considered the biological mother, and, thus, the only mother that the courts, schools, doctors, and the government recognize. Raye was not considered a parent, despite her genetic contribution.

For Raye to become a legal parent without endangering Ginny's status as the mother, she had to file for a second-parent adoption, the same process stepparents undergo. Second-parent adoption has given thousands of lesbian and gay families the legal right to cover their children on either person's insurance or to name them as beneficiaries in an inheritance. Courts in twenty-one states, including California, have approved second-parent adoptions. In late 1997, New Jersey became the first state explicitly to allow gays and lesbians to adopt jointly, as married couples do. Courts in Colorado and Wisconsin still disallow such adoptions. New Hampshire and Florida ban adoption by gays outright. But the discretion in most states, as in most adoptions, rests with the individual judge who can approve or deny the action. Raye and Ginny paid about $3,700 in fees for a home study, paperwork, and attorney fees to complete the adoption. The night before the home study, they were so nervous they felt sick.

The social worker who interviewed them in person and visited the boys filed a highly favorable report. Nonetheless, she felt she had formally to recommend against the adoption because there was no legal marriage.

Their attorney filed their case in a liberal California county. The judge they appeared before quickly approved the second-parent adoption, then posed for pictures with the family. The issue of a same-sex relationship never came up.

A friend's child asked, "Who is their dad?"

"Science," Raye said with a laugh. "Technology." Someday they plan to tell the boys about the donor and how they came to have two mothers, a Mama (Raye), and a Mommy (Ginny).

Their boys' grandparents plan to move to the United States because Raye's parents believe they will benefit from a daily male presence. The twins are accustomed to family gatherings: birthday celebrations at hotels, crowded Sunday brunches, noodles eaten on the twenty-ninth of every month to ensure a long life. They have often played pabitin. Ginny finds herself humming a tune her mother sang to her many years ago. She can't remember all the words, but she knows it is the right song.

18   Investing in the Future

The money gene fairly jumped in the family of Kevin. Carried silently to New York State by a poor County Clare man, it surfaced in the immigrant's son, who opened one of the first car dealerships in the eastern United States.

The money gene skipped the son who inherited the dealership—but turned up in his brother, who made a fortune in land speculation and the stock market. It skipped whole branches of the next generation, before emerging in the car dealer's seventh child, a blond-haired boy with his uncle's name and his intuitive understanding of money. Even as a child, Kevin could take it and talk it and make more of it than men twice his age, a talent as natural and inexplicable as luck.

At eight, he was already begging his uncle to take him to business lunches. As a college student, Kevin kept a suit in his car, always ready to go to any meetings. During his junior year in college, his mother died, and although his six brothers and sisters were older and more experienced, he was named executor of his mother's estate because of his knowledge of finances. He entered business deals, fraternity parties, and tennis courts with the same remarkable confidence and ease.

When he graduated college, Kevin's uncle loaned him $150,000 to buy an apartment building in Texas. The terms were strict: 10 percent interest due in five years. Kevin and his wife, Jennie, moved into a complex so lousy with drug dealers that he put his car in storage rather than leaving it in the parking lot. Their adjusted gross income was minus $17,500. They worked hard to turn it around. When they sold the building two years later, the couple left with almost $1 million cash and a thriving real estate business.

Brash, daring, and successful, Kevin was like his wealthy mentoring uncle in every way but one: He wanted a houseful of children, he wanted to make Jennie happy. By all appearances, Jennie was his opposite— quiet and reserved. In truth, his wife was his business partner and every bit as emotionally intense; she just carried it inside. She had grown up in a close family who never underestimated or mistook her, a shy woman's refuge. More than anything Jennie and Kevin wanted a family of their own.

It was a shock, therefore, when they learned Kevin lacked the sperm to do it. When Kevin and Jennie didn't get pregnant right away, he went in for a sperm analysis. His wife thought he was crazy; his father had nine children. His brothers were having kids. But, in fact, Kevin's sperm count and motility were poor, though his volume was about four times the normal amount. It was as though a cup of water was poured into each ejaculate, the doctor told him. His sperm were swamped. Kevin was devastated by the discovery. He and Jennie decided to go to a fertility doctor as soon as possible.

The couple had met on a California street while she was still in college. They shared a strong work ethic; both had started earning their own money in grade school. Both were natural athletes with a trust and reliance on the health and abilities of their bodies. Jennie played softball, volleyball, and tennis. Kevin played everything, including the stock market. He found a partner for whom that scarcely mattered. Money meant nothing to Jennie. Her idea of success was a strong family and the time to enjoy each other. Kevin proposed to her two years later, at the Statue of Liberty down on one knee. It was the Fourth of July. If she provided the quiet dignity in the relationship, he provided the fireworks.

In the early 1990s, fertility clinics had their own form of gridlock. The number of patients seeking help crammed into clinics waiting for appointments. Once inside, they didn't always get to see the doctor. Kevin and Jennie started making the rounds. In the end, no doctor ever said they could not get pregnant, just that their chances, statistically, were low. His sperm needed to be addressed. And they also learned the implications of Jennie's never having had a normal twenty-eight-day cycle in her life. Her cycles stretched from thirty-five to forty-five days, and many months she likely didn't ovulate. She had polycystic ovarian syndrome, a condition in which cysts developed in ovaries and affected ovulation.

Their first directive was to try intrauterine insemination. Jennie had a slight bend in her cervix, and the medical staff at the clinic the couple went to sometimes couldn't get the plastic catheter through it. Jennie would lie there, feeling a bit overwhelmed. She never complained during these procedures, but her body would flush a bright telltale red, betraying her inner pain. The couple tried—and failed—eight times. The doctor advised them to consider in vitro fertilization. Jennie never forgot what the doctor said next. She said, if you think this has been a roller coaster, you need to be prepared for IVF. Who would guess, Jennie said later, that she would be on that ride for years.

The doctor was right. Their first in vitro fertilization cycle in Texas, in October 1994, was a disaster. There was no fertilization. The second, two months later, resulted in two cleaved embryos and no implantation. Ditto for cycle three in March. When Jennie and Kevin moved west in 1995, they underwent cycles four and five. In both attempts, the clinic they went through was providing ICSI. They got eggs, they even got good embryos, but they didn't become pregnant.

As the years had passed, Jennie's two sisters and Kevin's seven brothers and sisters, and their friends had babies, many and often. Jennie and Kevin would get a phone call notifying them of another pregnancy; Jennie would be fine for a day or two, then the emptiness that overcame her swallowed any joy she felt. Family functions, baby showers, even birthday parties became strangely awkward.

One night as the siblings in Kevin's family gathered for dinner honoring his oldest sister, the circle of flushed faces and unity was so intense that Jennie had to excuse herself to go to the bathroom to cry. This was the magic and power of a family, she thought. One that for her and Kevin appeared to be out of reach.

Resiliency, though, was the gift from her parents. When Jennie faced the grief of the failed cycles, when even Kevin felt like they were not meant to have a family, Jennie would repeat a lesson her mother had always said, "Where there is life, there is hope."

In this way, the couple was able to go on. They went to one of the best urologists in the country, where Kevin underwent surgery to tie off a varicocele, an enlarged varicose vein in the testes that produces too much heat and may raise the temperature in the scrotum, thus affecting sperm. A varicocele can be asymptomatic, or can ache. In rare cases, if the vein causes chronically high scrotal temperature, the testicle may atrophy and, over time, shrink, causing sperm and hormone production to go down.

Jennie and Kevin bought a big, black dog. They went to Europe. They talked about adoption. But the more Jennie learned about open adoption, the less comfortable she felt. She was turned off by the idea of their having to sell themselves as parents to a potential birth mother. She was a private person and didn't want to open up their lives for scrutiny. Kevin, who could trace his ancestors back four generations on both sides, revered the idea of the family and heritage. Blood ties to him were sacred and unifying. But they were both running out of energy for more fertility treatment. A free fertility seminar was being advertised in San Jose, in the heart of the Silicon Valley, and they decided to check it out. She told him she had the emotional and physical strength for one more attempt. Jennie and Kevin's work ethic carried them to this point. To them, the job wasn't finished until it was a success.

The hotel conference room rented by our center held nearly four hundred people. Well-dressed couples in their forties, newlyweds, and same-sex couples come to these seminars. I had just finished my presentation and was standing at the podium taking questions on hyperstimulation when a long arm shot up in the middle of the room on my right-hand side.

A six-foot-six man stood and, in a clear, booming voice, said: "I'm zero for three. My wife is thirty, she makes lots of eggs, and I have a sperm problem. What could you do to treat us?"

"How old did you say?"

"Thirty. We did three cycles that didn't take, and we actually had two others that didn't even get to the transfer."

"You are the couple we dream about treating," I said. "Number one: Because of your wife's age. Number two: She is a high responder. Number three: We know good ICSI can bypass the sperm problem. Number four: We can check for an immunological problem."

"You're saying there is something you can do?"

"There is no reason why the two of you can't get pregnant," I repeated. "And your chances should be 50 percent each time we treat you."

The conversation goes back and forth like a tennis ball until he ended with what sounds like a challenge. "I'm coming in to see you Monday," he said.

Next to him, his wife is looking at me as though I'm trying to sell her a used car with an IVF option. Skepticism is all over her face. I can see her looking at her husband asking: "Who is this guy?"

When Jennie and Kevin's medical file arrives at my desk, it's nearly four inches thick. The dozens of blood tests, hundreds of injections and pelvic examinations it represents, not to mention the two surgeries, are testimony to the lengths this young couple has gone to try having a child. Most people would have run out of emotional and financial stamina long ago. Their costs have got to be approaching $150,000. Now I understand the look on Jennie's face. It's fatigue.

In a marathon, we call it "hitting the wall," reaching the point when exhaustion erects a barrier in front of a runner as real as one made of brick. Each step becomes a monumental effort that ends in pain. I can remember hitting the wall two-thirds of the way though the Comrades Run, the fifty-six-mile ultramarathon from Durban to Pietermaritzburg, South Africa. I was practicing medicine in a two-thousand-bed hospital in Kwazulu, the Zulu homeland, before the end of apartheid. The wall is where your body and mind are saying, "You are not going to go a step farther." For a time, you don't remember what happens next. Hitting the wall forces you to reach deep inside for the strength to keep going, because nothing outside is going to get you through. And for most people, lying down, which is the number one physical urge at that point, is not an option.

Jennie and Kevin have hit the wall in assisted reproduction. No one is encouraging them or giving them any energy to keep going. I need to try to help them to the end of the marathon. I just need to find the way.

After a couple has had five failed in vitro fertilization cycles, a lot of reproductive centers won't even accept them because working with a couple that doesn't ultimately bear children could lower the center's overall success rates. Others would treat Jennie only if she used donor eggs, saying that she has bad eggs. Looking at their chart before they arrive, I think that neither assumption is true.

A lot of young women are told that they have bad eggs. I've known twenty-three-year-old egg donors and women in their early thirties whom I've helped to go on to bear children with their own eggs who had been told previously that they had bad eggs, an opinion that needlessly crushes them and their hopes of ever having their own genetic children. Some young women do have "bad eggs," poor-quality eggs that make poor-quality embryos that may be chromosomally abnormal. But it is very rare for a woman to have poor eggs at age thirty. I don't believe we're looking at an egg problem with Jennie. It is more likely a stimulation problem in which the drug protocol prescribed for Jennie has failed to produce the most, and the most mature, eggs while eliminating the risk of ovarian hyperstimulation syndrome.

Kevin and Jennie do have a male factor, and despite his varicocele surgery, he still has a sperm count of 14 million with 16 percent motility. The ideal is 20 million with 40 percent motility. A good ICSI program will go right around that barrier. It doesn't matter if he has 20 sperm. So, our challenge, clearly, is Jennie.

The secret of a good stimulation will be the prolonged coast. Jennie has undergone years of shots and examinations. She was hyperstimulated once in a previous cycle at another clinic. She is young and has polycystic ovarian syndrome so will likely produce two or three times the average number of follicles. Jennie has already had a laparoscopy in another program, and we review the film in our office a few days after we meet. The diagnostic laparoscopy was normal, but it helps me to confirm her polycystic ovaries and, in addition, to see that her uterus is normal.

The first thing I need to do for them is arrange immunologic testing. I usually decide to take a couple after an initial consultation, if I can determine I have something to offer them. I'm prepared to take on a couple like Kevin and Jennie if we find something in the immunological testing that needs treatment. If we can find certain autoantibodies, for instance, we can neutralize them, thus eliminating another negative variable. On the other hand, if there is no apparent immune problem with this case, my staff and I are probably going to have a result similar to the other in vitro clinics. But the immunologic screening shows a clear problem. Jennie tests positive for four of eighteen antiphospholipid antibodies (APA) that we screen for, including two of those we believe affect pregnancy most. Phospholipids are the building blocks of cell walls, the glue that holds cells together, and they are vital to implantation and growth of the placenta. The antiphospholipid antibodies are autoantibodies that have long been linked to recurrent miscarriage. These antibodies can attack the membranes in the microscopic blood vessels of the early placenta. Our data suggests that to overcome this abnormal immune response, she'll need immunoglobulin, IVIG, prior to the transfer and at least once a month for the following three months.

I am also going to have her take twice-daily shots of heparin and a daily baby aspirin.

"Whatever it takes," she says.

Jennie and Kevin can afford to do more financially if this fails. But they must also be able to afford it emotionally. Jennie has been so taxed by the previous failures that she remains skeptical from the start, doubtful that there is anything that will help. But as they have throughout, they pull each other along.

Kevin is feeling challenged and invigorated. One reason Kevin was even interested in our seminar was because of the money-back guarantee we offered at that time. Like Kevin, most of our patients love it. Our critics and competitors hate it. Critics charge that we are guaranteeing a baby. But the first lesson I learned in fertility medicine is that I don't have the divine power needed to guarantee whether someone becomes pregnant and has a baby. I can only help make circumstances right for a pregnancy and pray that it happens. Our shared-risk program doesn't guarantee a baby; it guarantees people can leave a life crisis with their dignity and savings, and move on if their cycle is not successful.

Critics have also voiced their concern that the risk sharing on the center's part will change how we manage individual patient care decisions. This is a concern, certainly. But it is abhorrent to think that a patient's medical care would be influenced by their financial arrangement with our front office. Personally, I want to know that a patient is in the refund program only if they are in the 30 to 50 percent of patients for which a cycle doesn't work. The only reason I want to know then is that I feel better knowing that, if they leave without a baby, they will still have their equity intact to try again, or to move on with their lives. Kevin says he hopes, if anything, that the shared risk will lead to better care and attention to detail.

"I think doctors should be accountable just like every other professional in the world. When you buy something, you should get what you pay for, or get a refund."

As we plan the retrieval and transfer for early December, Kevin's oldest sister takes a turn for the worse. Eighteen months earlier, a stomachache Patricia complained of was diagnosed ovarian cancer. The family is thrown into the grief and helplessness of a catastrophic illness.

Kevin crosses the country shortly after we speak to be with his sister in the last weeks of her illness. He takes his telephone, fax, and laptop computer, and moves into his aunt's house. Typical of his traditional family role, he handles all financial questions surrounding his sister's illness and impending death.

Jennie starts the cycle while Kevin is away. She gives herself her own shots and, as November passes, travels to join her husband. Our center ships medication and syringes to cover her care while she is there. In the midst of the crisis, Kevin and Jennie decide to tell no one about their attempts to have a baby. Kevin's sister, Patricia, dies on Thanksgiving Day.

I am struck again by how many patients lose family members during treatment. Many of my patients are of the age at which their own parents are beginning to succumb to illness and old age. It is not uncommon for a couple to experience a death in the family while they are in the middle of their own crisis of infertility. Kevin has lost both parents and his oldest sister at very young ages—before any of them reached fifty-two. What a calamity that is. One of the reasons that we as human beings may want children is to be reminded that life goes on, renews, begins and builds again, and that we are all part of a continuum. How often the birth of a baby seems to follow a loss. Infertility robs us of this natural renewal of hope.

A week after the funeral, Jennie comes to the center to have the ultrasound scan of her follicles. Jennie mentions that she's grateful that she and Kevin operate their own business, in their home, or she doesn't know how she would get the time off work to undergo all the testing. She will start her first intravenous immunoglobulin infusion, a three-hour procedure, that week.

Our tests show that Jennie is responding so well to the fertility drugs that, on cycle day eight, we are ready to discontinue the medication and initiate the coast, withholding any more drugs and coasting her until her estrogen levels drop to a safe enough level for us to administer the hCG shot. Three days later, her estrogen drops, and she is ready. On the day of the retrieval, we retrieve thirty-two mature eggs. It's a great response, and her fertilization rate is even better: twenty-six eggs fertilize with ICSI, an impressive 81 percent. Normally, 70 percent fertilize.

This is a woman characterized as having an egg problem—yet she has gorgeous eggs that yield nineteen healthy embryos after being mixed with Kevin's sperm.

Before the transfer, we need to make decisions about the number of embryos to put back. With her excellent response and fertilization rates, they are feeling hopeful but still cautious. The average number of embryos to put back in a woman her age is three to four. But Jennie, with five unsuccessful attempts behind her, is hardly average. I will probably suggest they consider four.

When we discuss the numbers, I can tell her that she has a 50 percent chance of pregnancy, and, once pregnant, there is a 40 percent chance of a multiple pregnancy—a 34 percent chance of twins and a 6 percent chance of triplets or more. I recommend four. But if we are going to transfer four, they need to understand the risk and be able to consider selective reduction.

Jennie knows it is their decision. They are desperate to have this happen.

"You've taken us this far, we'll go with what you recommend." We transfer four embryos.

That December was grayer than usual, and the air off San Francisco Bay is bone-chilling. Jennie and Kevin couldn't seem to get it together even to Christmas shop. They weren't shoppers anyway, but they felt even less like it with the loss of his sister Patricia still so recent and raw.

Jennie is home alone the day the telephone rings. "Jennie, this is Anna from PFC," Anna Hosford says. "Are you sitting down? It's great news. Your tests indicate that you are pregnant at this time."

Kevin is at the gym playing basketball, and, when she reaches him, he cries and will cry every time he thinks of that conversation. In three days, it will be Christmas. He tells her, "We don't need to buy presents. We have everything we want."

It is overwhelming. They'd never had good eggs; this time they got so many that we are able to freeze fifteen embryos for future use. They'd never been pregnant; now they are. In fact, her blood tests suggest she is carrying more than one, and it soon becomes clear it's a major multiple. They are nervous and expectant and can't wait until the first ultrasound.

It is a major multiple. All four embryos we transferred have implanted. Here is this couple who has come to us for a baby after years of failure. That four would implant and survive is completely unlikely, and yet, it happened.

Many times nature will self-select and some gestational sacs will vanish. But Jennie and Kevin are soon forced to make a choice. They reduce to twins. No matter how much we discuss the possibility before the transfer, when it comes down to it, selective reduction is one of the most difficult things to proceed with. They go back and forth for days, torn between what they'd like to do and what is best. In the end, they make the right and most difficult choice, for the benefit of Jennie and the unborn twins.

Postscript

"What reduction?" the genetic counselor asks them several weeks later. Jennie had undergone amniocentesis, and on the basis of the results, Jennie and Kevin were asked to come in to speak to a genetic counselor. Driving into the meeting, they were heartsick with worry. Jennie, as usual, was trying to think positively. But she was also determined; she knew that they had gone too far and they would accept and gratefully love any child they got.

The geneticist sketched a large chart of family history of illness and deaths and talked for nearly an hour. At one point Kevin said something about the multiple pregnancy. That's when the counselor blurted out that she didn't know about the other embryos. Apparently, the medical group interpreting the amniocentesis results did not treat the pregnancy as a multiple, and thus the results suggested major health problems with the twins. Once adjusted, the numbers were normal. After the longest hour of their lives, Jennie and Kevin returned home.

The pregnancy continued healthy and normal. Jennie walked regularly and swam right up to the end. At thirty-eight weeks, she delivered Michael, five pounds and Patrick, seven pounds, seven ounces, and named after Patricia. And they both believe that he looks like his auntie. His brother, people always point out, looks just like Kevin.

That is our goal for each cycle, a single healthy baby, or, at most, two. Jennie and Kevin have two healthy children. The babies take naps late in the morning. Jennie, who has been working since 5 A.M., runs up the stairs at the couple's home when she hears them stir. She opens the blinds, singing, "You are my sunshine," and the warmth in that room doubles. She holds her babies, sometimes carrying them down the stairs, all twenty-five pounds of them. Her life is complete. She calls to Kevin, who leaves his desk in the middle of the workday to meet his wife and partner in the kitchen, where she is fixing applesauce and noodles for lunch. She watches him bend his long form and sing. Kevin recently had a chance to take over a very lucrative property out of state, but it required extensive time away from home—away from Jennie, and their investment in their future, their twins. No way, he said, swinging Patrick in the air.

19 On-line

$\mathcal{D}$isease is often silent. Before it is ever detected, a single infection from a sexually transmitted disease can damage a fallopian tube. Endometriosis can build pelvic adhesions silently for years, gradually pulling the organs in a woman's abdomen apart or binding them together again, unnoticed. Such conditions often become obvious only by their result: infertility.

Likewise, the pursuit of the diagnosis is often silent. The failure to conceive was, for years, the burden between the couple alone. Few people outside the relationship knew the reason they did not have children. Infertility was inferred, never stated as obvious. Miscarriages were not discussed or acknowledged. Women didn't know anyone who shared their problem. The silence created its own set of symptoms: depression, anxiety, guilt, isolation, and, sometimes, suicidal thoughts. This was much of the landscape until the mid-1990s when the personal computer became, for infertile couples, a personal friend, a guide, and a community.

On the Internet, women in rural Wisconsin could go to the website for the National Library of Medicine and read *The Lancet* or *The New*

England Journal of Medicine. They could visit the Centers for Disease Control or their doctor's office. They found national organizations and recently published research, and legal opinions on surrogacy, egg donation, and assisted reproduction. But, most important, they found one another.

In the fall of 1995, Hilary Sachs, a professor of French and linguistics at Columbia University, was trying to have a baby. She knew that there were other women like her—professional women in their forties who had postponed childbearing to focus on their careers, but she didn't personally know anyone in her situation. She'd had two miscarriages in less than two years since her marriage at thirty-eight. Sachs was lonely and needed someone to talk to, someone who was going through what she was going through. She would find herself on the World Wide Web looking for information and support. It occurred to her that she could organize a group that created a safe and supportive environment for women like her. Starting with a series of E-mail messages, she founded Fertility^{SM}, a members-only on-line support group. Within two months, Sachs knew forty-five women, all subscribers, who shared her concerns, hopes, and her fertility problem. Within two years, she knew almost four hundred.

Diana was one of them. An accomplished classical musician turned computer systems analyst, she had succeeded in arena after arena in her life. But a series of long-term relationships had ended without marriage or children. The men she dated were either not right for her or not interested in children. Up until age thirty, she figured it didn't matter. At about thirty-four, she began to realize how much it did matter. She had always wanted kids. Her twin sister's daughter called her "my other Mommy." She loved that word. *Mommy.*

Diana met David, a law student, through a personal ad. Since they married when he was thirty-nine and she was forty-one, she'd been living, breathing, and typing infertility. Specifically, alt.infertility, and Fertility^{SM}. Diana had visited a gynecologist and begun taking clomiphene when she discovered infertility resources on the Internet and got an instant education. Sitting before her glowing computer screen, she learned about uterine lining, fertility drugs, and why women over forty shouldn't wait for a full year of trying (as was frequently advised) before getting aggressive. "Get moving" was the general advice she received on-line, and, not long afterward, Diana did. The decision that it takes many people six years to reach, she and David reached in six months.

That fall, Diana was turning forty-two, she and David began an in vitro fertilization cycle, just nine months after they officially began trying to have a baby. They knew from their reading that Diana was a human hourglass, monthly losing irreplaceable ovarian time. The problem they had to overcome, the doctor said, was "old eggs." David's sperm count, motility, and morphology appeared to be just fine.

In August 1996, they began an in vitro fertilization cycle. Diana's ovaries produced eleven eggs. But the next day they learned only two had fertilized. Up until then, they had never really had bad news in their pursuit of parenthood. This was bad news. They knew from their extensive reading that one of the only ways to increase an older woman's chances for a baby was to increase the number of embryos transferred.

David had arranged a series of telephone consultations with different doctors whom they located on-line. One doctor asked if her husband, David, was taking high blood pressure medication. Yes, Diana said, a calcium channel blocker. David had been on it since he was thirty, she reported. That's when Diana and David realized that the medication he took every morning may be affecting his fertility. Though his sperm looked fine, they probably weren't penetrating the egg, the doctor surmised.

I was one of the doctors they consulted that week. I spoke to them on the car phone on a Tuesday night as I was driving home across the Golden Gate Bridge. They said they were in the middle of an IVF cycle—their two embryos were being transferred the following day—and they had experienced poor fertilization. They asked if being on a calcium channel blocker could be having an effect.

I told them that the law of unintended consequences is that medication to improve health in one area may be detrimental in another. Nowhere is this as obvious as in fertility. Chemotherapy and antibiotics, such as sulfa drugs, can kill sperm. High blood pressure medication, including spironolactone, can affect how sperm function. Alpha blockers, such as phenoxybenzamine, prazosin, and ganglion blockers, affect ejaculation.

I tell Diana and David that there is an association between calcium channel blockers and low or no fertilization because the drug may prevent the calcium shift necessary for sperm activation. Calcium is needed for the acrosome reaction, the activation of the tiny cap on the sperm's head that releases enzymes. The reaction is the critical point when the warhead of the sperm becomes armed for penetration, as opposed to being covered and protected. I faxed them two medical journal articles the next morning describing this effect.

After reading the material I had sent, Diana was surprised and excited when their doctor called ten days after the couple's two embryos had been transferred to report that her pregnancy test was positive. She was told that her beta test results were 30, right in the middle. Diana and David immediately called their parents and friends. Two days later the doctor phoned back to say there had been a mistake—the blood had been tested for progesterone, not for the pregnancy hormone. Diana wasn't pregnant.

Diana and David were crushed—and angry. The doctor had never mentioned the problem with the blood pressure medication, though it was clearly recorded on their medical chart. They set about trying to recoup the money they spent and renewed their efforts to start another in vitro fertilization cycle with a different doctor.

David went to his family doctor, who easily switched him to a different high blood pressure medication, an ace inhibitor. They contacted the author of the articles I'd faxed them, who said it would be at least ninety days before David's body regenerated the sperm cells enough for the couple to have any chance of a natural conception. Diana, who felt like she was watching the doomsday clock in ovarian time, didn't want to wait.

They call me, and I schedule our work to begin the week she'll turn forty-two. I was optimistic that we could help her and David become pregnant.

Two months after our initial conversation, David and Diana come into the office. David is fairly stressed, he's preparing for his state's bar examination. Diana is calm and clear about what she wants to do. Bouts with a blood disorder in her teens, and ulcerative colitis in her thirties, have turned Diana into a smart health consumer, and she can discuss her treatment in a very objective, intense way. She is a no-nonsense person. She has no problem with the fertility drugs and no patience with people who do.

Diana has also been pregnant before. Shortly before they were married, she and David had conceived and miscarried. This episode alerts me to test Diana for antibodies that may increase the couple's risk of miscarriage. I tell them we can also do assisted hatching to ensure the thick membrane of the fertilized egg is sufficiently weakened to allow hatching and implantation. But our biggest and clearest weapon to overcome the egg-sperm problem is ICSI.

Before a woman begins a cycle through our clinic, I require that she undergo a hysteroscopy, a direct examination of the uterus. Many people protest that it is an unnecessary and costly step. But we've found unforeseen problems in one in seven women we screen. Diana is one of them. There is a spiderweb of scar tissue in her uterus, most likely due to the previous miscarriage, that could interfere with implantation and cause another loss. The obstetrician who performed the hysteroscopy scheduled a dialation and curettage (D & C) to remove the spiderweb of tissue in Diana's uterus, and three weeks later, we started them on a stimulation cycle.

When Diana and David come in for the transfer, we get very good news. They have three embryos, not a lot, but the quality is superb. Two of the three are excellent, divided with six and seven cells. Normally, we expect 10 percent of embryos to be flawless. Two-thirds of her embryos are. Diana only has three embryos, which, in some ways, makes the decision about how many to transfer easier. We'll use all three.

On December 9, Diana learns from our staff that her pregnancy test is positive. She and David are thrilled and are leaving for a trip to New York to mark their first anniversary and celebrate.

But in the airplane bathroom, Diana discovers blood. When she calls me, I tell her that a number of women have implantation bleeding after a procedure and that it may be especially obvious when a woman is taking blood thinners, such as heparin and aspirin, as Diana is. I ask her to call us if anything further develops. Two days later, she calls the office again from a New York City hotel room. She has abdominal pain and when asked to describe it on a scale of 1 to 10, she says this registers a 20. I tell her that she needs to see a doctor immediately. A pregnant woman complaining of abdominal pain should always be aware of a possible ectopic pregnancy.

The pain is so extreme that Diana goes to the emergency room in an ambulance. An ultrasound shows two gestational sacs in the uterus, and a faint shadow on her left side. The one sac looks empty. The other has just the beginnings of a fetal pole, the collection of developing cells that will become the whole baby. It is still too early to see a heartbeat. Doctors theorize that Diana has an ovarian cyst that is causing the pain and that the bleeding is due to the imminent loss of the smaller sac. Diana is given pain relief and sent home. The next night she and David go to Carnegie Hall to watch her sister, a classical musician, perform. Afterward, the pain returns in waves, and David takes her back to the hospital. The second trip to the doctor reveals nothing new. On December 30, when she returns to San Francisco, she comes into our office to have an ultrasound to confirm her pregnancy. Her face is alight as we watch the screen together, the little embryo is already growing and changing, but I also see the shadow on the left side, and I tell Diana that we need to keep a close eye on that. Her pain seems to be continuing intermittently, and I want to watch her progress closely.

The next day, as the whole world prepares for New Year's Eve revelry, Diana calls our answering service, desperate. The pain is so bad she can barely stand up. I admit her to the hospital and schedule a laparoscopy. I'm going to go in myself to have a look.

When I see her and David at the hospital, Diana is completely deflated. Having to go in for abdominal surgery that requires an anesthetic, she has no illusions that any baby will make it through alive. I try to reassure her that the chances of losing the uterine pregnancy are slim. But she has had life experience otherwise that makes her doubt my words. Mentally, she's trying to imagine and focus on her next IVF. The last thing she says before she goes under anesthetic is that if she can just see the next plan of attack, she's sure she can get through this whole thing.

Through the laparoscope, I can clearly see she had an ectopic pregnancy of eight weeks on the left-hand side. The fallopian tube looks like a snake that swallowed a golf ball. It appears bloody and is fixed behind the ovary and uterus. The pain had to have been intense, I say aloud. The fallopian tube is swollen from the middle to the fimbriae end, and appears stuck between the large bowel and the back of the uterus. It was apparent to me that there was a blood clot organizing that was causing the pain she experienced in New York. The tube is not ruptured, but the end is bleeding. Left untreated, this could rupture. We caught it just in time. Ectopics can turn the joy of a pregnancy into a nightmare so easily—they still kill healthy young women every year because we miss the signs and symptoms.

In fertility medicine, the unintended consequence of transferring embryos into the uterus is that one or more can wander into the fallopian tube. It probably happens more times than we know, but since the embryo fails to implant and grow, it goes undetected. But when you have a pregnant patient with vaginal bleeding and abdominal pain like Diana's, you almost have to assume it's an ectopic pregnancy until proven otherwise.

I'm able to remove the mass and her tube through the laparoscope. I remove the tube to prevent an ongoing or persistent ectopic growth of tissue that could jeopardize Diana's uterine pregnancy. The whole procedure takes about forty-five minutes. Afterward, when Diana is recovering, I'm happy to tell her that the surgery went well and the little one growing in her uterus appears to be doing fine.

We hope that, when the incisions heal and her tummy feels better, she can begin to relax and enjoy her pregnancy. The failure of her previous IVF and now this complication are the things that I often see rob a woman of her ability to enjoy this miraculous time. I hope this doesn't happen to Diana. Two weeks later, in my office, we review the videotape of her laparoscopic surgery together. The baby she so feared losing is growing nicely. At twelve weeks, we send Diana and David on to the care of her obstetrician.

Postscript

Danielle Marie is born at five-pounds-plus on August 15. She has her father's coloring but her mother's eyes. From the get go, she appears petite, tough, and a bit noisy. It's pretty obvious who she belongs to.

The first clue something was wrong after the birth, though, was when Diana asked a friend who had also just delivered, "When do your ankles stop hurting?"

"Your ankles hurt?" the friend said.

From two days after delivery on, every joint in Diana's body hurt. She often felt nauseated, weak, and exhausted from nursing the baby every three hours. She didn't even want to tell the doctor. "Well," she imagined the doctor saying. "You wanted a baby." Her doctor did say, "Look, you're forty-two years old."

She was eventually hospitalized with a diagnosis of endometritis or a uterine infection and was treated with oral and intravenous antibiotics. Several weeks later, Diana E-mailed me that she was still having pelvic pain. The Internet has given me a whole new way to communicate with my patients. Although my typing has never improved, with a voice-activated computer, I'm able to quickly share information through E-mail or my web page, www.GoIVF.com. As a rule, I do not diagnose a patient on-line, but I know Diana and I needed to know if her doctor had considered whether there might be placental tissue still in the uterus. The most common reason for acute infection after childbirth is that the woman has retained tissue.

I tell Diana my suspicions and tell her that she needs someone to look and see. I refer her to Dr. Camran Nezhat, a specialist at Stanford University, for a laparoscopy. Almost four months after the birth, he found placental tissue in the uterus that had not been removed during her cesarean section. It was causing a chronic infection. Dr. Nezhat performed a D & C. Diana called several weeks later to say she was improving.

She and David are thrilled raising Danielle. The baby is toddling and learning to talk. Her first words were "quack, quack" and "dada."

Often, late at night when the baby is asleep, Diana will creep downstairs to the computer and log on to the Internet. She still regularly joins infertility discussions. She isn't seeking information so much as catching up with friends. New people join every day, and she wants to offer a little advice and hope, as people did for her before she and David had Danielle.

Two years after Hilary Sachs helped bring such women together by founding Fertility[SM], she became pregnant herself naturally and delivered a son. On-line, one learns that there are many paths to parenthood.

20 A Mother's Love

People who work the graveyard shift don't get enough sleep. Neither do the mothers of infants. So Dorothy was getting a double shot of sleep deprivation in the winter of 1958. She cared for her nine-month-old daughter all day, then went to work every other night at the hospital where she was a nurse. Graveyard shifts were quiet but hardly uneventful. Dorothy cared for patients with pneumonia, cancer, and broken hips. She must have walked ten miles a night. Now she was pregnant again with her second child, and it felt, well, a little soon. She was tired.

Her first child was just at that oh-so-perfect and plump stage, fat cheeks and toothy smiles, always drooling; she was so sweet. It was wonderful to see, especially since at birth she looked like a little old stick person. The pregnancy had gone a month past due to almost forty-four weeks. Nowadays doctors would recognize placental insufficiency and they'd induce a baby like that and let her mother bring her home. But in 1957, they let you go and go, and so Dorothy went and went. By the time the baby was born, she was so sickly they didn't think she'd pull out of it. She weighed just over five pounds, and the doctor thought the baby girl was probably taking nourishment from her own body tissues because the placenta was failing.

For this baby, her second, Dorothy was seeing the best obstetrician in town. Her dearest friend from nursing school had gone to work for him, so she knew she was getting good care. She'd had no trouble with her first pregnancy, and she hadn't suffered much discomfort with this one, never a moment of morning sickness or bleeding. She'd never had a miscarriage. She was just tired. During a routine visit, the obstetrician said he was going to start Dorothy on some medicine that might make for a fatter, healthier baby, and Dorothy said fine.

But the pills made Dorothy sick, nauseated. She would go to work, and if a patient was vomiting, she was practically vomiting on top of him. She knew she couldn't work feeling that way. So she compromised. She took the pills every other day, on her days off. Toward the end of the pregnancy, Dorothy's husband took a job in another state, so her obstetrician never saw the result of his prescription on her newborn. In fact, it would be years before he did. Dorothy delivered a five pound, six ounce baby girl on a July night. They named her Hannah.

Dorothy had been an only child who became close to her own mother only as an adult. In fact, growing up she had received more attention and warmth from the maid than from her own mother. She wasn't going to do that, and she and her husband built something rare for their two daughters: a house of confidence and trust and love. Dorothy was a born worrier, so she worried about her kids' health and safety. But she never had to worry about Hannah. Hannah always filled her in; she shared her secrets.

She was, her mother would say, the easiest kid in the world. Hannah loved school, loved to read, loved other kids. You could never take her anywhere in a hurry, because Hannah couldn't walk down a street without stopping to speak to every child she saw. She was president of her class and of practically every club she ever joined. She was homecoming queen. When Hannah graduated high school, her principal said she should have worn roller skates to the ceremony because she had to come to the stage to collect awards so many times.

But all those accomplishments came later, years later. Years after Dorothy's husband walked into the kitchen carrying an article in a medical journal about a drug called diethylstilbestrol, DES. It was a synthetic estrogen prescribed for more than thirty years to prevent miscarriage. When taken by women in the first five months of pregnancy, it caused birth defects in the reproductive organs of the children being carried.

In females, it caused changes in the cells and structure of the vagina and uterus. Some baby girls were born with a uterus the walls of which were distorted; others had a little hood on their cervix. All were at increased risk of vaginal cancer. Male babies' testicles didn't descend or were unusually small. It was a scientific and pharmacological catastrophe that would, among other things, increase the risk of breast cancer in the women who took it. The federal government estimated 5 to 10 million people were exposed to DES during pregnancy and effects would eventually be detected in the third generation. To top it off, DES didn't even prevent miscarriage.

Today when people get an unfamiliar prescription, they pull down the *Physicians' Desk Reference* and look it up, Dorothy thought. But people didn't question things in 1958; they just didn't. People assumed that if the doctor prescribed medicine, then there was no question that taking it was safe and advisable. Dorothy's husband said she shouldn't feel guilty for doing what the best doctor in town said to do. But the destruction caused by DES was so awful that there was no way around it; Dorothy picked up the burden of association. She would always feel sadness, guilt, and the deepest desire to turn back the clock and throw away every single one of those pills.

Dorothy and her husband, Don, immediately did what they could to monitor and mitigate the possible effects of DES on their daughter. They took Hannah to the best gynecologist in town, possibly in the state. He was going to examine Hannah every six months for effects and to watch for cancer that developed in women exposed. The specialist was not gentle. He was not patient. When he roughly put his hands in Hannah's vagina, she would flinch. He would say, "Don't be such a sissy." When her mother said, "Do you have to do it that hard?" he said, "Don't be such a nervous Nellie." Hannah was eleven years old.

When she was twelve, a major DES clinic opened up in a city nearby. Dorothy accompanied Hannah to her appointments, where the staff was gentle but the exams no less invasive. Through it all Hannah never cried.

Nor did she dream. She had no illusions in high school about falling in love and pushing a baby carriage. She did not suffer a gross physical abnormality from the DES as some did, such as a double uterus, that would have made it obvious she couldn't have children. Doctors were still learning about the effect of more subtle differences, such as the shortened cervix that she appeared to have. Nevertheless, Hannah felt she could not dream as other girls could. The appointments made it clear, even to her young mind, that her reproductive organs were so flawed they required constant monitoring. Doctors were looking for vaginal adhesions, cancer, and any changes. As a teenager, she didn't know anyone else who had to undergo the humiliation and invasion of these gynecological examinations. After her first gynecological examination, Hannah left the office saying she never wanted to marry. She was naturally good with children and longed to work with them and have children of her own someday. But she suppressed those feelings and started looking for a career into which she could throw her energy and intellect. She went to business school and began work toward her MBA.

But life is unpredictable in so many ways. She met Charles at school. He was warm, loving, and optimistic. They were married.

It was the early 1980s, and Hannah was on the corporate fast track, living on the East Coast and working sixty-hour weeks. She'd begun having pelvic pain, which her doctor diagnosed as endometriosis. He warned that if she ever wanted to try to become pregnant, she ought to try soon, before the endometriosis worsened. Hannah would be forever grateful to the man. She'd always used birth control, and she and Charles decided they would try to see if she could become pregnant. It was then, at twenty-six, that she did. Motherhood was a certain career ender, but Hannah and Charles were thrilled. This was what she felt born to do.

Hannah was in her sixteenth week of pregnancy when her doctor discovered her cervix was 85 percent effaced, or thinned in preparation for labor. Her quick-thinking physician performed an emergency procedure to insert a stitch in her cervix and ordered her to bed. Nearly half of such emergency sutures fail.

Dorothy dropped everything and crossed the country to be there and help her daughter. She took care of Hannah's needs and helped her daughter to be able just to rest. When Charles took a job at a firm near Hannah's parents' home, Dorothy packed up their house and moved them into her and Don's house to complete the bedrest until the baby was born. Dorothy set Hannah up in her guest room and put a typewriter near the bed where she worked on graduate-school papers. Dorothy and her husband waited all night in the hospital waiting room when Hannah delivered at thirty-six weeks.

In the delivery, Hannah's placenta pulled away from the uterus after thirty hours of labor. Her blood pressure dropped so low she was in mortal danger. The doctor had a hard time getting the bleeding to stop.

Dorothy and her husband were in the waiting room gripped with trepidation. When a healthy boy was born, Hannah and Charles named him after his father. Hannah fully recovered from the ordeal. Despite occasional worries about having stepped off the corporate track, Hannah was happier than she'd ever been. Eventually Hannah went back to work, and Dorothy got the opportunity to care for the baby. The two women were good friends as well as mother and daughter. They were both nurturers and nesters. They spent hours companionably in each other's company. Dorothy loved seeing how natural and contented her daughter was with the child.

Then, when the baby was ten months old, Hannah and Charles were offered positions three thousand miles away. It was a career opportunity for both of them. But in the restored quiet of her own house, Dorothy was sadder than she'd been in a long time.

After her son was born, Hannah never used birth control again, hoping to become pregnant once more. When she finally did become pregnant at age thirty-three, she miscarried. She spent five years of her life between the ages of thirty-three and thirty-nine trying to have another child. She traveled across the country twice to try different treatments. If a doctor had told her to lie in bed for five years to have a baby, she'd have happily jumped into bed. But bedrest wasn't enough. For five years she took injections of fertility drugs. She became pregnant and went in to have the cervical stitch put in. She asked the doctor why he didn't do an ultrasound first. No, he said, we'll do it after. So he inserted the stitch. And the ultrasound afterward showed that the baby was dead. Hannah was grief-stricken and angry at the toxic exposure that she believed was the cause. In her life, DES had always been there, like an ominous shadow. But after she married happily and had a son, she had slowly begun to believe that she might have a normal life, despite the DES. But now the old ghost was back and more malevolent than she could have imagined. She would become pregnant and the babies would die because of the structural weakness in her cervix caused by DES. For years, she and her mother and father had spoken about DES in medical terms and physical results, and not about the psychological toll. But now, the cost was too great. In her grief, Hannah lashed out at the unfairness of the world and all the people in it, including sometimes even her mother. Hannah had never blamed her mother; she just thought her mother was too trusting and too good-hearted. Hannah did blame the doctor. She began to hate that doctor who had given her mother the DES. She pictured screaming at him. She felt deformed. She felt like she was not enough of a woman to carry a baby.

Dorothy watched her daughter's anguish helplessly. When Hannah was on bedrest during a pregnancy, all Dorothy could do was travel to her and begin working, making soup and doing a hundred small things to make her daughter comfortable. Her heart was in her throat the whole time.

Hannah became pregnant again on fertility drugs, and this time the stitch held. It held right up until her membranes broke at sixteen weeks and the nourishing and nurturing fluid the baby was floating in dropped hour by hour until the baby was dead. The memory of it will haunt Hannah for the rest of her life. She thought, The poor little thing. . . .

Hannah went to a place so blue and hopeless that her mother could not reach her. Her wonderful joie de vivre gone. She began to set her sights higher for her career and prefaced many sentences with: "Since I'm not going to have any more children . . ."

Dorothy and Don encouraged the couple to adopt. They were ready and able to take off to a country like China at any time to assist them with an international adoption. Hannah was ready, too, but Charles hadn't reached that step.

When the couple moved back west again, they bought a house within a few blocks of Dorothy and Don's. That Christmas, when Hannah made ornaments as she always did with her growing son, it became clear he was maturing beyond some of his childhood traditions. It was devastating to see how fast he was growing up. Hannah counted up the years remaining and realized she'd be only forty-four when he went to college. There would be no more handmade ornaments, no more children for these traditions.

Dorothy and her husband had seen articles and a few television programs on surrogacy. Suddenly, to them, the arrangement seemed to make perfect sense in their daughter's case. Another woman could carry an embryo created from Hannah's egg and Charles's sperm. She had to tell Hannah.

Dorothy was trusting. She had always believed in altruism, unexplained kindness, and that people usually meant well. Even when she thought back about the physician who had prescribed the DES, the memory conjured up more sadness and guilt than anger at him. Dorothy thought the doctor was a nice man who meant to do the right thing. She felt comfortable suggesting surrogacy to Hannah, because she and her husband truly believed that there was someone loving, giving, and strong enough to carry a child for their daughter. Charles agreed.

Hannah thought her mother—and her father and husband—were crazy. Why, she asked them, would a woman carry someone else's baby? She had seen a lot of conniving and even untrustworthy people in her career and dealings with the public. She was also living with the consequences of vast, medical betrayal. She thought that anyone involved in surrogacy was probably sick, doing it for money, or both. Hannah told her husband and parents that she was sorry, but she didn't believe in altruism. She'd just spent the last fifteen years in corporate America.

But Dorothy and her husband and Charles all begged her at least to reconsider. Hannah needed a professional opinion on the matter, and she felt as if she had to resolve any lingering questions about her own fertility. That's when she called me.

Of the several hundred couples I see a year, a small percentage are DES-exposed, but they leave an impression. At the beginning of my work with every couple, I take a family history and ask specifically whether either of the couple's mothers had any history of miscarriage or took any pills during her pregnancy. Many DES-exposed people have no idea they were exposed until they experience infertility. They never knew because their mothers didn't remember or were never told. Hospital records and physician records often disappeared or were destroyed before it could ever be confirmed. Often the proof of DES exposure is obvious during a hysterosalpingogram, an X-ray examination in which dye is injected to see the shape of the uterus. The DES-related abnormalities can also be detected during a hysteroscopy when I directly examine the uterus and cervix while the patient is under anesthetic. Normally, the cervix protrudes into the vagina like a little nose. But in a

DES daughter, it is a little flatter than it should be; it may even be flush with the vaginal vault. It can also have a little hood on it, known as a cock's comb, where the cervix is shaped like a rooster's comb with a red vascular appearance. The walls of the vagina also may have a polyplike appearance or rawness.

In DES daughters, the uterine cavity is often small and may be configured in a T-shape. In some women, the walls of the uterus are closer to each other than they should be. So that instead of looking into a triangle when I look into the uterus, I'm looking down a narrow tunnel, with barely enough room for implantation and growth. Many of these structural abnormalities of the uterus or cervix can lead to miscarriages or preterm birth. The fallopian tubes in a DES daughter can have a wider-than-average opening, predisposing her to ectopic pregnancies.

Many DES daughters are able to conceive readily, but they also experience higher rates of miscarriage and preterm birth. The children of DES who reach me are more often like Hannah, devastated by multiple losses or years of infertility. DES is among medicine's worst legacies. But there is hope; DES does not appear to affect the ovaries or eggs. Today I'm meeting Hannah to talk about gestational surrogacy.

Hannah is here in the office with her mother, Dorothy. Charles is working and so Dorothy volunteered to come along to support her daughter and keep her company on the drive into San Francisco. The two women are on a fact-finding mission to investigate Hannah and Charles's options. I have the privilege of speaking with both women as the three of us sit down together in my office.

DES has created many victims, the first of whom is the woman who innocently and trustingly took it. Hannah is overcome with emotion as we begin speaking, but I can see the anguish also in her mother's face. I think of how I feel, as a parent, whenever my children feel pain. To know that your actions may have played a role in something as damaging to a child as DES is almost inconceivable. You suffer as your child suffers. I have spoken to a number of mothers who have beaten themselves up for years and years over DES. Like most women, Dorothy took DES without knowing what it was. She was told that it would help her have a healthier pregnancy. Other DES mothers have told me they believed they were taking a vitamin supplement. Yet even this truth does not ease the pain these women feel.

I tell Dorothy that she has carried a terrible grief about this and that she must understand that it wasn't her fault. Dorothy starts to talk and acknowledge how badly, how truly awful, she has felt over the years. Her burden only increased with time, of course, because of Hannah's miscarriages. For Dorothy, there is no question that our discussion has reopened a terrible wound. She spoke about her pain and wept. But I am also trying to give her the space to forgive herself, just a little. I tell her the pain and anguish will always be there. It just changes a little with time. I'm hoping that, by acknowledging the guilt and worry she has lived with, both she and Hannah will begin to heal.

We talked about Hannah's pregnancy history and what her options are. By the end of our conversation, I believe that Hannah is finally coming to terms with surrogacy as a choice. But she makes it clear this is not an easy conclusion for her to reach. She feels as if giving up carrying a baby is giving up too much. I tell her to take some time, think about it, and call me. I hope to see Hannah and Dorothy again.

It takes several months for Hannah and Charles to contact a surrogacy agency. Charles is excited by the idea, as are Hannah's parents. But Hannah still has doubts. She is skeptical even as she and Charles find a potential surrogate, a young woman who has served as surrogate before and has children of her own. Hannah is skeptical right up until she meets Donna. But when the two women meet, they click, instantly, over lunch. Donna agrees to help them. Someone at the agency asks Donna why she is going to help Hannah and Charles, a couple who already has one child. She said because of the extent and length of their grief. She is so calm and has such an aura of decency that Hannah finds her doubts disappearing.

Hannah telephones me, and we launch a cycle that spring, using Hannah's eggs, mixed with Charles's sperm, and transferred into Donna's body. Even as the procedure progresses, as we retrieve ten eggs and transfer six, Hannah remains skeptical that a pregnancy may result.

But it does. Donna is pregnant. When she and Hannah come into my office four weeks later for an ultrasound scan, Hannah brings her mother, who meets Donna for the first time. Dorothy instantly clicks with her as well. As joyous as the news of the pregnancy is, I realize that the stress Hannah is feeling is peaking when I see her face at the ultrasound scan. She is terrified of miscarriage; she had been so traumatized by her own that she figures this pregnancy will end, too. She is afraid to even look at the monitor. What if the worst happens again?

I can only be calm and reassuring. The ultrasound scans continue to show a healthy ongoing pregnancy. Donna is in terrific shape. The baby grows and grows. Dorothy prays and prays. Every other week, she takes an advertisement out in the *San Francisco Chronicle*, giving thanks for the intervention of St. Jude, the Catholic patron saint of lost causes.

Postscript

Hannah and Charles were in the room with Donna when their baby was born. It was a boy. Their entire extended family crowded into the room almost immediately after. Donna watched in pride as Hannah and Charles held their baby, Christopher, crying tears of joy and relief. Hannah looked at the woman who had given them this gift. She admitted it aloud: Her parents were right. There is goodness in this world that is inexplicable and miraculous.

Hannah and Charles took the steps necessary to formally and legally adopt their son and bring him home to join his older and beaming brother. Hannah took the baby to visit Grandma Dorothy and Grandpa Don almost every day. Dorothy and Hannah delighted in the baby's every development, spending many companionable hours together.

A few months later, the telephone rang at Grandma's house, and it was Dorothy's dearest friend from nursing school. She was in town with a friend and wanted to get together for dinner. Her friend was the obstetrician who gave Dorothy DES.

Dorothy then revealed what her experience had been with the doctor and the pain that the DES had caused in her daughter's life. She talked about the lost children, the betrayal her daughter felt, and her loss of trust in the world. Dorothy said if the couple still wanted to come to visit, she would be happy to have them to dinner. But she said she was going to call Hannah and invite her, too. The friend, and the doctor, said they wanted to come.

Hannah went straight to her mother's house as soon as she got the call. She helped her mother prepare the meal, and together they set the dinner table, as they had for so many years.

That night the doorbell rang, and it was Dorothy's friend and the doctor. Dorothy hadn't seen the man in forty years. Hannah had seen him in her mind every day for as long as she could remember. She hated him.

The gentleman, well into his seventies, moved to clear the air as soon as he entered Dorothy's home. He told Dorothy that she was one of two women to whom he prescribed DES. They told him how it had affected Hannah, the baby she had been carrying. As the evening progressed, he asked Hannah to forgive him. It was the last thing that either of the women had expected to hear. When I learn of the dinner later, I think of how rare and remarkable that encounter was. I can only think it eased their grief and gave them the ability to continue to heal. But the baby was the sweetest salve.

In the months after the birth, Dorothy did two more things: First, she wrote to the surrogate, Donna, and thanked her for the gift of life. Second, Dorothy and her retired husband took over care of the baby while Hannah went back to work two days a week.

Sometimes Dorothy wonders about the couples she saw in our waiting room on her visits accompanying Hannah. What happened to the young woman in the red jacket? The couple who wanted the baby so badly? The man in the Levi's at the computer? She'd like to tell them what happened to her: a grandson; a daughter healed; and peace.

21 Second Opinions

Consider the lesson of Leslie, who was told at age forty-two to retire any hope of having her own children. "It's probably not going to happen," the doctor said. "You really need to think about opening yourself up for disappointment. If you want to be a parent, you need to keep adoption in mind."

The special education teacher practically beat herself up on the drive home from the appointment. Why hadn't she and Michael tried to have children earlier? The question of children would come up, and life would push the conversation away. They married late, when she was thirty-four, and there was always a sense they were just getting settled. Plus, she had the example from her own history. Her mother hadn't had her until age forty-one.

Even when she was younger, doctors had warned Leslie that she might have trouble conceiving because of polycystic ovarian syndrome (PCOS). Each month, the follicles, the small bubblelike sacs that hold eggs in Leslie's ovaries, would begin to mature normally. But then no single dominant follicle would emerge to release its mature egg. Instead, over time, small cysts formed in the ovaries. Leslie would go six months without a period. When she did have a cycle, it didn't necessarily mean she had ovulated. Over time she developed fine hair on her upper lip—a sign of abnormally high levels of androgens, the hormones responsible for male characteristics. The PCOS also increased her risk of developing acne, heart problems, uterine cancer, and diabetes.

With age and anatomy against her, Leslie visited her doctor and began taking the synthetic hormone clomiphene in March 1995. The drug works by causing the pituitary gland to increase the amount of FSH secreted, thereby stimulating follicles to grow. Leslie continued the drug until September without getting pregnant. Her doctor referred her to a fertility specialist in northern California, who prescribed fertility drugs and artificial insemination, saying that they had a 4 percent chance of success each cycle.

In late December, a blood test indicated Leslie was pregnant through intrauterine insemination. The couple was so excited. Four days later, Leslie started spotting and then bleeding. January 2, the first day back at school in the new year, she spent the day at home. She had miscarried. They tried with one more cycle, but it was canceled because of hyper-stimulation.

It was a dreary, depressing time. Michael, a corporate communication specialist, regretted not trying earlier and began gauging their finances to chart their next course of action. As a child, relatives had given him stock for presents on birthdays and holidays. He cashed in the stock. Leslie saved nearly $1,000 a month from her teaching salary for a year. It was enough to try an in vitro fertilization cycle.

Leslie looked at the money they'd gathered and felt some fear. They weren't gamblers; they'd never even been to Las Vegas together, and on their one trip to Reno, Nevada, they stuck to the quarter slot machines. They didn't even know if they'd be accepted for treatment at an in vitro fertilization center.

When they contacted our center, the doctor said that Leslie had probably passed the point of being able to be a genetic mother, that her best chance of taking home a baby probably lay with egg donation.

"If you choose to try with your own eggs, our clinic will do it, but your chances of becoming pregnant are so incredibly low it would be like throwing a basketball out a fourth-floor window and making a basket across the street," the doctor said.

Leslie and Michael looked at each other. They wanted children. They decided to take the shot.

On May 19,1996, she began a cycle. They had nine embryos available for transfer, the doctor said, but they were heavily fragmented. Based on her age and the quality of the embryos, the doctor advised transferring all nine. He also recommended against their trying again with her own eggs. The embryos were transferred. None took.

Over the summer, Leslie thought about their lives. In her job, she worked with children whose problems ranged from significant developmental delays like autism to mild problems with comprehension and retention. She found constant joy in how children saw the world. She and Michael decide they want to try to adopt. They called a well-known adoption attorney and arranged an appointment—he had no openings for five months and required a deposit to hold the appointment. They sent the $600 deposit in and, once again, sat back to wait.

But Leslie couldn't stand how their medical journey had ended. She felt like she had left the in vitro process with unresolved feelings and some complaints. If their dream of a genetic child was over, Michael and Leslie wanted closure, some sort of endpoint, so they could move on. That's when they called me.

Lesson Number One: If you are thirty-seven or older, and planning to have a baby, you've lost ovarian time just reading this.

Michael and Leslie are here in my office to review their failed cycle and past treatments. When I look at their file, all I can see is red. Physicians have taken one of Leslie's most priceless possessions—her ovarian time—and they've wasted it.

Leslie was forty-two years old when she started seeking help to have a baby. It is an outrage to prescribe repeat doses of clomiphene to a forty-two-year-old woman when success rates are so low and the time left on the ovarian clock is so fleeting.

For mature women, anything short of the most aggressive approach wastes time.

I do not recommend clomiphene at all for women over the age of thirty-seven. On the one hand, it can and does prompt the ovaries to make multiple follicles. On the other hand, it can also compromise the quality of the mucus in the cervix and antagonize the lining of the uterus to the point that it is not receptive to implantation, a side effect that can last as long as six to eight weeks.

In a young woman who makes large numbers of follicles and eggs, those consequences can be counterbalanced by her vigorous estrogen response. As a woman gets older, the downside starts outweighing the potential benefits.

I also tell Leslie and Mark that I recommend strongly against staying on clomiphene for more than three cycles because, in my experience, 85 percent of couples who benefit from that regimen will do so within that window of time.

The single most important predictor of whether a woman can successfully have her own genetic child is the age of the egg.

Women over thirty-seven who want to have a baby should go straight to their doctor for complete reproductive testing, including a hysterosalpingogram, an X-ray to determine the condition of the fallopian tubes; blood tests to record baseline levels of follicle-stimulating hormone and estrogen; a base immunological antibodies screen; and a semen analysis for her partner.

Fortunately, it is not too late for Leslie and Michael. If there is anyone who can become pregnant at forty-three with her own eggs, it's Leslie. Because she has polycystic ovarian syndrome, I tell her, the source of her infertility may very well be the source of her solution.

Normally, a woman's ovary is about the size of a California walnut. As she nears ovulation, her follicles appear on an ultrasound monitor as dark fluid-filled bubbles. In a natural cycle, one of those follicles will mature, ripen, and release a mature egg. In a stimulated IVF cycle, many follicles will mature, and the doctor can retrieve many eggs.

A polycystic ovary such as Leslie's is two to three times larger, even in the resting phase. Women with PCOS often speak of a dragging feeling or a sensation of heaviness in the pelvis. They've often been told that it is their imagination. But polycystic ovaries are markedly different, covered with a thickened capsule and filled with small fluid-filled follicles. Through the laparoscope, the polycystic ovary, which does not release the egg easily and regularly, has a smooth and pearly white appearance. There is a conspicuous absence of the pits and scars of past ovulation.

Leslie's eggs are older and forty-three-year-old eggs are more likely to have abnormal chromosomes; they make fewer healthy embryos and have a smaller chance of growing into a healthy baby.

In PCOS patients, we can balance this natural decline in quality by sheer numbers. Because of the syndrome, I'm expecting that Leslie will produce two to three times the number of follicles expected for her age. She'll also require less fertility drugs.

I tell the couple that the biggest bugbear that Leslie faced earlier—hyperstimulation—is not an issue, because our technique of prolonged coasting will eliminate the risk of developing severe ovarian hyperstimulation syndrome while allowing us to retrieve a good number of mature eggs. We can also add heparin and aspirin empirically to improve implantation. I'm also going to recommend assisted hatching, to help an embryo implant.

Leslie and Michael really need to go home and consider their options. Is it going to be adoption or another IVF cycle? I've told them how I try to get the message out: Women with PCOS have the highest chance of success with IVF of any patients in their age category.

On the drive home, Leslie notes the appointment with the adoption attorney is still months away. They could do an IVF cycle with me much sooner. This is a gamble, Michael says, but the payoff could be exactly what they want.

On July 28, she begins the medication to suppress her ovaries and then begins a series of fertility drugs. I've prescribed a level of drugs usually aimed at much younger women because I know she'll respond well—she does. By the third week of August, ultrasound examinations and blood tests reveal that dozens of follicles have responded, each now measuring nearly three-quarters of an inch.

On the morning of August 23, we retrieve twenty-five eggs. After the eggs are mixed with Michael's sperm, we get thirteen embryos. The quality of the embryos is slightly better, and they are dividing much better than before.

The day before Leslie turns forty-four, we plan to transfer the embryos that have fertilized and grown. Leslie and Michael come in that morning, and we meet to make some decisions about how many to transfer back to her uterus.

As women age, their eggs age. The result is that fewer and fewer are likely to fertilize, implant, and grow into a healthy baby. The chance of a woman becoming pregnant in one cycle with her own eggs when between the ages of forty-three and forty-five is 10 or 12 percent. Her chance of becoming pregnant rises with each additional embryo transferred, but the age and chromosomal normality of the eggs likely negates some of that gain. As I tell all older patients using their own eggs, we generally need to transfer up to four times the number of embryos into a woman at forty-four that we would have needed when she was thirty, and we will still have less than a 30 percent success rate. So in order to come anywhere close to those results with Leslie, we need to transfer all thirteen.

We also know that the chance of a multiple pregnancy in women over forty also goes down to less than 10 percent when using their own eggs. The risk of triplets would be 2 percent. Leslie and Michael understand, and we proceed to the transfer.

On September 5, when Leslie comes home from school, the results of the pregnancy test are on the answering machine. They were so eager to know they told our staff to leave a message if they were not home. The message said, "The results indicate you are pregnant at this time." Leslie immediately runs out for balloons.

At week six, at the ultrasound, there are two gestational sacs. There's a heartbeat and then, moments later, a second one.

"Is that a second one?" they both ask.

My partner tells them yes. "But please don't be surprised if the next time you come one of them has disappeared." He explains the syndrome of the vanishing twin since the second sac appears smaller. Leslie feels almost a sense of loss.

"I am going through a grieving process," she tells a friend. "I'm happy, but there is a part of me that sees that little sac, and I think, That's a person who's not going to make it."

At week nine, she goes in for the ultrasound, afraid that neither fetus has survived. She knows that more than 40 percent of all pregnancies in women aged forty to forty-four end in miscarriage.

On the ultrasound screen, one sac and heartbeat is obvious and nicely developed since the last exam. So is the second one. It seems to have rebounded and caught up.

Leslie and Michael are so elated they buy a disposable diaper that day, wrap it in a box, and deliver it to Michael's mother. "Guess what?" says the card inside. They are so excited they finally send out a pregnancy announcement. It is a Far Side cartoon by Gary Larson, depicting a dog, pedaling a unicycle on a high wire while juggling balls, hoops, and a cat. The caption reads: "High above the hushed crowd, Rex tried to remain focused. Still he couldn't shake one nagging thought: He was an old dog and this was a new trick."

Postscript

A month later, Leslie developed gestational diabetes. The obstetrician described it as garden-variety diabetes, but she needed to take it easy. She'd always worried about how healthy she would be during a pregnancy, but it was a happy and relaxed time. At thirty-six weeks, she had a C-section because the babies were transverse. They were boys weighing five pounds apiece, Joseph and William.

Leslie laughs that already she has been mistaken for the boys' grandmother—twice. But she and Michael say they feel reenergized and delighted by their sons.

Which brings us to Lesson Number Two: Miracles do happen. They're in the playpen right now. "That's the yardstick for all miracles," Michael said.

Conclusion:
What's New in IVF

The ability to fertilize egg with sperm outside the human body has changed the face of human reproduction forever. Since the birth of the first IVF baby in 1978, more than 300,000 children have been born through assisted reproduction. We can now remove eggs from one female to help another achieve pregnancy. We can remove sperm directly from the testicle, allowing men to father a child who would otherwise not be able to. We can inject a single sperm into an egg to promote fertilization, virtually eliminating severe male factor and failed vasectomy reversal. We can transfer the gametes of one couple to a host uterus, allowing implantation and pregnancy to occur. The technology of manipulating gametes has become more sophisticated. From injection of a single sperm (ICSI), we have now moved to the molecular level where we are removing the nucleus and shortly individual chromosomes and genes from reproductive cells.

The newest breakthroughs in assisted reproduction include a renewed focus on the mind/body connection to fertility; advances in genetics, including preimplantation genetic diagnosis (PGD), stem-cell research, cloning, and gene therapy; as well as advances in storage, specifically the storage of eggs and ovarian tissue.

The Mind/Body Connection

Western medicine has traditionally been resistant to alternative therapies, focusing on the management of disease after it presents. Alternative therapies and traditional medicine in many cultures focus on the whole person, and they generally ask questions about causation and methods of prevention. Traditional Chinese medicine consists of acupuncture and herbal therapy to treat and prevent disease. This effective form of medicine has been practiced by almost a quarter of the world's population for 5000 years. Evidence of Traditional Chinese Medicine (TCM) treating infertility dates back to 11 A.D. Ignoring lifestyle, diet, exercise, and the power of the mind has forced patients to choose between alternative therapies and Western medicine instead of combining the best of both worlds.

Mind/body medicine combines modern scientific medicine with psychology, nutrition, exercise, and stress management. I believe in the connection between the mind and the body and the beneficial effects of aligning these for optimal results with our fertility treatment.

Research has shown that women experiencing infertility have higher levels of physical and psychological symptoms, which could include (but are not limited to): insomnia, headaches, back pain, fatigue, anxiety, and depression. These symptoms may affect the embryo's ability to implant successfully through abnormalities detectable in the immune system. A recent study demonstrates that patients undergoing IVF, who already have higher scores for anxiety, also have abnormalities measurable within their immune systems. This group of patients had lower implantation rates and lower success with IVF compared to patients who were less anxious and were found to have fewer disturbances of their immunological systems.

Mind/body techniques are aimed at helping to reduce stress and promote positive attitudes. I urge my patients to look into alternative services such as acupuncture, Chinese herbs, and yoga that may reduce stress and calm anxiety, allowing them to regain the balance that has been lost in their struggle with infertility.

Acupuncture

Recent medical research has shown that acupuncture can improve the outcome of Assisted Reproductive Techniques (ART) by improving ovarian response and uterine receptivity. Currently there are two published acupuncture protocols, or treatment regimens, being used to treat infertility. The Swedish protocol requires eight acupuncture treatments, twice a week for four weeks, beginning the month prior to the transfer of the fertilized eggs. The more recently published study of the German protocol requires two acupuncture treatments at the time of embryo transfer—one appointment is scheduled the day before embryo transfer and the other is scheduled the day of or the day after embryo transfer. The German study showed improvement in IVF outcome when two sessions of acupuncture were added on the day of embryo transfer. The pregnancy outcome improved from 26 percent to 42 percent in the 80 patients surveyed. Many patients choose to combine the two protocols for maximum benefit.

Chinese Herbs

Acupuncture and Chinese herbs work together like surgery and anesthesia; one supports the other. Herbs have always been an integral part of Chinese medicine and play an important role in the physiological mechanisms involved with the uterus, hormones, egg development, and general health when preparing for pregnancy and during pregnancy. Herbs may also be important in helping to prevent miscarriage. It is important that the patient consult a licensed practitioner who has the proper training to know which formulas are beneficial and appropriate and which herbs are not.

Hatha Yoga

Another approach to mind and body is the practice of Hatha yoga, which promotes physical as well as emotional well-being, assisting in the alignment of the mind and body. Hatha yoga can also be extended to include meditation as well as visualization techniques, which have been shown to decrease stress and the release of stress hormones, thereby creating an optimal environment for implantation.

In general, I encourage all my patients to examine their habits and lifestyle, paying close attention to the elimination of unhealthy behavior such as smoking or inappropriate alcohol consumption, while evaluating diet, exercise, and the effects of stress on their health. We have all heard of the epidemic of obesity in our society, and the resulting mortality and morbidity. In addition, recent evidence shows that obesity affects fertility by promoting hormonal imbalance and problems with ovulation and implantation. **Body Mass Index (BMI)** greater than 30 for any recipient will decrease IVF success rates by 50 to 75 percent. This applies to conventional IVF as well as egg donation and surrogacy. Studies have shown that nutritional supplements such as antioxidants, multivitamins, and amino acids can enhance egg and sperm production, leading to better fertility outcomes. For additional information please visit www.fertilityblend.com.

We encourage patients to evaluate the mind/body connection in every step of the fertility process—before IVF is initiated, at the time of embryo transfer, and after successful implantation has occurred. Therapies that do not address the whole individual—including their genetic predisposition, their environmental exposures, and their lifestyle choices—are destined to achieve less than optimal results. We are just beginning to appreciate the concept of wellness and to realize the power of the mind over the body in all facets of our daily health, especially in the area of fertility. By holding Eastern and Western medicine as complementary, rather than mutually exclusive, we can enhance the standard IVF treatment cycle to produce maximum results.

The Genetic Revolution

The successful race to map the human genome has spawned faster computers and methods of genetic analysis, as well as phenomenal interest in using this new information to better understand, prevent, and treat disease. Applying this knowledge to the embryo will alter the way IVF is practiced and the future of reproduction.

PGD

New technologies like Preimplantation Genetic Diagnosis (PGD) allow genetic testing to be completed in a shorter time and on ever-smaller samples of DNA. Currently, children born in the United States have a 3 to 4 percent chance of a major birth defect. Some of these abnormalities occur because of a single-gene defect that is inherited from one or both of the parents, while other abnormalities are related to **aneuploidy,** or an abnormal number of chromosomes. We'll look at both conditions in more detail, but generally PGD permits the selection of embryos that are less likely to have chromosomal abnormalities and also embryos that may be free of a known single-gene disorder—thereby increasing the likelihood of a healthy baby and decreasing the chances of having to terminate a pregnancy found to be abnormal. Chromosomal abnormalities in embryos are responsible for a significant proportion of failed implantations after hormonal, uterine, and immunological factors have been excluded.

Couples in which the woman is 35 or older can use PGD to test for age-related chromosomal disorders, or when there is a single gene defect within a family. The majority of PGD procedures are performed for abnormalities in the number of chromosomes, and this problem increases with increasing maternal age. Studies have also shown that up to 85 percent of aneuploids are caused by the egg, while the sperm may cause the remainder. When PGD is performed for aneuploidy, unfortunately we cannot check for single gene defects at the same time unless more than one cell is removed from the embryo.

Younger women with repeated unexplained miscarriages can also benefit from PGD. Even in "optimal situations," in which the egg provider is under age 30, the percentage of embryos that have normal chromosomes may only be approximately 50 percent. PGD procedures help doctors select and replace only those embryos that appear to be normal, so that women may increase the chance of conceiving while reducing the probability of losing the pregnancy or carrying an abnormal baby to term. PGD for aneuploidy can determine the presence or absence of certain numerical chromosomal disorders, and PGD for single gene can detect certain genetic diseases but cannot predict congenital malformation.

Females are born with all the eggs they will have in their lifetime. As a woman advances in age, her eggs are exposed to aging processes that include chromosomal abnormalities. Thus, the chance of conceiving a chromosomally abnormal baby increases with age. In contrast, sperm are newly made every 65–75 days, so the risk of chromosomal abnormalities due to paternal age is much smaller.

Chromosomes are stringlike structures found in the center of the cell, the nucleus. Chromosomes contain genes that are made of DNA, the molecule that contains inherited information. Normal human cells contain 23 pairs of chromosomes, a total of 46. We receive 23 chromosomes from each parent. If an error occurs leading to the egg or sperm having an extra or missing chromosome, the embryo created by that egg or sperm would have an extra or missing chromosome (aneuploidy). If the aneuploidy involves chromosomes such as 13, 18, 21, X, or Y, the pregnancy may still carry on until birth, even though the fetus has a chromosomal disorder. Trisomy 21 produces an effect called Down's syndrome. The effects of other common aneuploidies include Turner's syndrome and Klinefelter's syndrome. These disorders are nonfatal, in that the fetus can carry to term and result in a live birth, although the baby is abnormal. Overall, the risk of aneuploidy is known to increase with maternal age, from 1/385 at 30, 1/179 at 35, 1/63 at 40 and at the age of 45 the chance of delivering an affected child is 1/19.

In addition to aneuploidy, there are now more than 60 single-gene diseases that can be diagnosed with PGD. Most of these genetic syndromes are relatively uncommon, and doctors classify them as either dominant or recessive. Dominant defects are transmitted by one parent alone, with the risk to the affected child being 50 percent (e.g. Myotonic Dystrophy). Recessive defects occur when both parents have the gene with the risk to the affected child being 25 percent (e.g. cystic fibrosis, sickle-cell anemia, or Tay-Sachs disease).

The preferred method of PGD is to remove one cell from an embryo on Day 3 of development; at this stage the embryo usually has 6 to 10 developing identical cells, each with a full complement of chromosomal material. The embryos remain in culture while the cell is analyzed. Normally, only a single cell is removed from each embryo, as it is expected to be identical to all the other cells, but it may be necessary to remove a second cell according to circumstances. In either of the above cases, the analysis of the biopsied cell uses a technique called Fluorescence In-Situ Hybridization or FISH, which takes about one day. The cells are fixed to a glass slide and heated and cooled, and their DNA is "labeled" with colored fluorescent dyes called probes, one for each chromosome analyzed. At present, the test can check 9 chromosomes out of 23. Once the FISH procedure is complete, the geneticist counts the colors using a powerful microscope, thereby distinguishing normal and abnormal cells. This information is then related to the normalcy of the associated embryo being held in culture. After this process the biopsied and analyzed cells are no longer viable in any way, and the slides on which they sit are discarded.

There are new strategies now available that allow analysis of all 23 chromosome pairs. A procedure called Comparative Genomic Hybridization (CGH) is now available but requires 2 to 3 days for complete analysis. This amount of time requires that the biopsied embryos be frozen and transferred in a subsequent cycle. When considering the losses associated with freeze/thaw survival of biopsied embryos this procedure is not currently practical. New CGH protocols are being developed that reduce the analysis time and this will allow us to test all 23 pairs of chromosomes and transfer fresh embryos.

Embryonic Stem Cells

Embryonic stem cells or master cells are *totipotent*, meaning that they have the ability to make any cell or tissue in the body. The ability to produce and harness these cells holds tremendous promise for transplantation and gene therapy and the elimination of many degenerative and debilitating diseases.

Embryonic stem cells are derived from the inner cell mass of the blastocyst and, if isolated and cultured in the laboratory, have the ability to develop into any cell in the body. Through the use of these embryonic stem cells we may one day be able to perform transplantation using only ultrasound guidance and a needle to inject the cells into the desired location. We may no longer require organs from people dying in tragic circumstances, as long as we can unravel the method of directed development in these stem cells to produce specific cell types or organs. Patients with spinal cord injuries may benefit from direct injection of these cells, which would then facilitate repair of spinal cord tissue. Diabetes affects almost 15 million Americans, and a simple injection of appropriately directed stem cells may be able to cure this devastating condition.

Embryonic stem cell research raises ethical questions because of the various methods of obtaining or producing the cells. Given that the cells originate in an embryo, any research involving destruction of an embryo may be totally unacceptable to certain people who would obviously also be opposed to discarding embryos or abortion or selective reduction.

The logical method of obtaining stem cells would be to use the thousands of embryos presently stored by fertility programs throughout the United States. Many of these embryos are destined to be destroyed because their owners have either completed their families or have decided to abandon treatment. IVF programs should discuss stem cell research with patients as an alternative to destruction when embryos are first stored. These embryos are an extremely valuable resource for preventing and treating disease and they should not be discarded if at all possible.

Another method of obtaining stem cells could be the creation of embryos specifically for the purposes of stem cell production, but this seems unnecessary in the light of the large number of embryos that already exist in storage.

A third and more controversial method of creating embryos for stem cell research is cloning or somatic cell nuclear transfer, which would create an identical genetic match for a particular individual requiring stem cells for disease treatment or prevention. This, in my opinion, is the most valid reason to support ongoing cloning research and it is unfortunate that the controversy surrounding creation of identical individuals impacts cloning research to generate genetically matched stem cells.

Somatic Cell Nuclear Transfer (SCNT)

Somatic cell nuclear transfer (SCNT), or cloning, has become controversial given the efforts of some to promote the creation of genetic copies of individuals. This controversy and debate detracts from the more important benefit of SCNT, which is the creation of stem cells that are an identical genetic match for a particular individual, enabling the treatment of disease and the alleviation of suffering.

Working in animals, and starting with Dolly the sheep, adult cells have been harvested and the nucleus removed and inserted into a donated egg from which the nucleus had been removed. This is somatic cell nuclear transfer. Subsequent to the birth of Dolly, many other animal species have been cloned successfully.

We should clearly make a distinction between SCNT and merely splitting an embryo, which happens naturally when identical twins are formed or when an embryo is merely cut in half, resulting in truly genetically identical offspring. When an adult cell has its nucleus removed and placed inside the donated egg, the resulting clone—while nearly identical in every way to the adult supplying the nucleus—carries some of the metabolic characteristics of the donor egg and the possibility of metabolic disease of the donor.

The experience gained from cloning animals tells us that the process is very inefficient, requiring many hundreds of donor eggs, most of which do not make embryos. Even when embryos are formed, most do not progress, and even those that do progress have a high risk of miscarriage once they are implanted into a receptive uterus. This method can also result in major abnormalities in embryos that do implant and grow, causing miscarriage or even severe medical complications for the carrier.

There are scientists and individuals who feel that we are ready to proceed with SCNT in humans, some for the treatment of infertility and others for aspirations of immortality. Looking at the animal data, I think we should exercise extreme caution. Cloning opens the door to a whole list of scientific, ethical, and moral issues, most of which we have not begun to address. Would cloning affect the health of the recipient mother or the health of the offspring? Is there a greater risk of congenital abnormalities? Will cloning adult cells accelerate the process of aging in cloned individuals? Ethical issues are also raised, relating to the uniqueness of each individual and the unrealistic expectations that we might place on cloned individuals. These concerns have prompted governments to enact legislation and also place moratoriums on human cloning until further research has been completed in animals. Unfortunately, the clandestine rush to clone humans threatens to derail the legitimate research that could result in cloned human stem cells being created with the potential of alleviating suffering and preventing disease.

Haploidization

A variant of cloning called haploidization may allow for the creation of an egg that could be fertilized with a partner's sperm when the egg provider is no longer producing healthy eggs. The female patient's somatic nucleus would be removed and inserted into a donor egg. During chromosomal division the genetic material is segregated, creating an egg containing half of the chromosomal complement of the female patient's somatic cell and capable of being fertilized with a sperm.

Haploidization is an attempt to avoid the pitfalls of traditional cloning. Reports on this procedure are preliminary and untested, but may offer hope to patients who no longer produce healthy eggs.

Geneticists are skeptical about the ability of the donor egg to completely reprogram the adult nucleus to become a healthy embryo, but this has not stopped the cloning of Dolly and other animals, or the clandestine groups who have claimed to have successfully cloned and delivered human babies who are apparently normal and healthy.

Gene Therapy

Gene therapy and germ cell transplantation hold promise for the elimination of genetic disease. While several strategies are being considered, the ability to perform gene manipulation on a germ cell removed from the testicle or ovary and then replacing it may allow the affected individual to then produce healthy eggs free of genetic disease.

Future Storage

Storage of Unfertilized Eggs

Cryopreservation, initially of sperm and subsequently of embryos, has been a major addition to fertility management. This process allows men to store sperm, often for 20 or 30 years, and then become fathers with the availability of intracytoplasmic sperm injection. This procedure is particularly attractive to men who are about to undergo chemotherapy or surgery. In addition, embryos produced during IVF have been stored, allowing patients to return years after their initial procedure and have another embryo transfer. This can result in a new sibling born from the same cohort of eggs many years later.

Women are born with all the eggs that they will ever have, and these eggs show decreasing degrees of normalcy with increasing age. On the other hand, men appear to produce sperm of good quality almost throughout their lives. Freezing unfertilized eggs when a woman is in her prime reproductive years, probably between 16 and 28, would seem like the logical way to preserve reproductive options for women, allowing them to compete on an equal footing with respect to education and career opportunity while maintaining their choices.

Unfortunately, there are some major problems with the freezing and thawing of eggs. Up to 500 million sperm may be available in a single ejaculate, but most woman only produce 10 or 15 eggs, even when stimulated with injectable medication. And obtaining the eggs from a woman is a more complicated procedure, requiring a minor surgical procedure called transvaginal egg retrieval. In addition, the egg is in a very delicate genetic position, and the damage from the freezing process renders most thawed eggs unfertilizable. The number of babies born from frozen thawed eggs is less than 50, representing a very low chance of success for a tremendous effort.

There is ongoing research into finding the best stage at which to freeze an unfertilized egg and also the best method of freezing and thawing. The ability to store eggs when they are in their prime will certainly level the reproductive playing field and narrow the gender gap that exists when it comes to procreation.

Storage of Ovarian Tissue

Because of the difficulties noted above with the freezing and thawing of eggs, scientists are exploring other options. One alternative being developed is the freezing of ovarian tissue. This operation has been performed in primates—the ovarian tissue is harvested, frozen, thawed, then transplanted back into animals. The result has been the production of follicles and eggs.

This technology holds tremendous promise for many patients, and possibly also for young women looking to store their eggs while still in the optimal window for reproduction. Many young women are faced with the diagnosis of cancer, requiring heroic treatment to achieve a cure, and many of these treatments unfortunately render the ovaries and their primordial follicles inactive. Ovarian tissue transplantation has already been performed in a young woman. One of her ovaries had been removed at age 19, and when the remaining ovary needed to be removed, pieces of tissue from the ovary were frozen. Subsequently, this tissue was thawed and sutured into her pelvis, and she appears to be able to ovulate when stimulated with fertility medications. There are risks, though—when ovaries are removed in the presence of cancer, there is always the concern that one could reintroduce malignant cells when the frozen tissue is thawed and transplanted.

Transplantation of ovarian tissue from one woman to another is probably not beneficial. As in all organ transplants, the recipient would need to take immunosuppressive drugs so that her body would not reject the foreign tissue. These same drugs may make a healthier pregnancy impossible. This means that transplantation of ovarian tissue will primarily be of benefit to a patient storing her own ovarian tissue for later use, either because of cancer or as a means of beating the biological clock.

A Final Word

Having been involved with IVF for more than eighteen years, I have experienced most of its growth and performed more than 9,000 egg retrievals. IVF started out as a controversial procedure available to very few, with a low rate of success. It has become a routine treatment protocol with ever-increasing success rates.

Most of the improvements we've experienced have taken place in the embryology laboratory, directly related to advances in technology. And it seems the future holds even greater promise with the advent of the genetic revolution.

We must always remember that IVF, like all treatments, is more successful when we work at achieving peak physical and mental condition. The connection between the Mind/Body and fertility cannot be stressed enough. The removal of toxins like smoking, alcohol, and stress from our lives; attention to diet and exercise; and the achievement and maintenance of an optimal BMI give us the edge we need to fight the best fight.

I look forward to continuing my work with IVF patients from all over the world and admire the courage and commitment they bring to their battle with infertility.

I wish you all great success.

Christo Zouves, M.D., currently resides in San Rafael, California, with his wife and two children. In December of 1999, Dr. Zouves realized a dream with the establishment of Zouves Fertility Center, located just south of San Francisco in Daly City, California. Believing that age, marital status, relationship arrangement, or financial situation should not limit any one individual from being treated, Dr. Zouves provides the latest treatments with the most technologically advanced techniques in his state-of-the-art facility. To learn more about Dr. Zouves and his team, visit his website, *www.GoIVF.com*, or contact his office directly at (800) 800-1160.